BY THE CUSP OF THE MOON

BY THE CUSP OF THE MOON

Finding Hope & Healing Beyond Suicide

D. R. Fredi

BY THE CUSP OF THE MOON

Copyright © 2019 by D. R. Fredi

For information contact :

http://www.SuicideFree.org

Book and Cover design by Dani Alcorn

ISBN: 978-1-7330308-2-3

First Edition: August 2019

10 9 8 7 6 5 4 3 2 1

We read to know we are not alone.

~ C. S. Lewis

Contents

PREFACE

FIVE YEARS HAVE PASSED since Jack took his life. We were married almost 20 years and yet, I still didn't know him. I would never have imagined that he, regardless of his ups and downs and eccentric nature, would choose to leave us, and all he'd built, but his mind got the best of him.

Most of us struggle at times with sadness and despair. Life is hard sometimes. I get that. And while I would never condone suicide as a solution to anything, there's a part of me that certainly understands the depth of despair that could cause a choice like this. After nearly 3 years of Jack's health spiraling downward, I understand the pain can be so intense nothing is worth staying in the game of life.

When he first began talking about taking his life, I lived each day with the hope, or idea, I could change his mind. Or maybe it was more that I didn't believe he would actually do it. I thought maybe it was a ploy for attention or just drama in the moment. Moments dragged on to days, weeks, and months and I managed as well as I felt I could.

I share my story not because I want to bare my personal life to the world, but because Jack dreamed I would write a book to help others struggling with the same issues. While our outcomes weren't what we hoped, I learned so much about loving with vulnerability, transparency, and as unconditionally as I could. I also learned I could not control what was out of my circle of influence and that radical acceptance is not an empty concept. Accepting what is or what has happened, or simply accepting I cannot control decisions made by others is imperative to my own mental health.

I loved Jack. I have no doubt Jack loved the kids and me the best way he could. The fact he took his life doesn't diminish that. While I would not have chosen for him to leave, I now understand why he had to and I don't fault him for it.

He was diagnosed with a bipolar condition, which was possibly complicated by some sort of attachment disorder but nothing was ever confirmed. Jack may have been... just Jack. He was an enigma in his own right. There were very few people in the world who understood him—and he liked it that way.

He saw the world differently than most people do. Undergirded with exceptional intellect, he had the ability to wield words in a way that would dazzle the most accomplished intellectuals. I have memories of endless conversations we had on subjects I hadn't ever discussed with anyone else. We would banter for hours. He was the first man to really hold my attention in a casual conversation. Jack's expansive interests made him a "jack-of-all-trades" in a sense. His grandmother once told me, "The problem I see with Jack is that he's good at everything and a master of none. He won't settle on just one direction because he doesn't have to."

He was well educated and well read. He knew things about which I hadn't a clue. Mesmerized for hours, I listened intently to stories of history, physics, medicine, and politics. We had conversations deep and rich.

Some say the gauge for intelligence is the sense of humor. Playing on ordinary environmental cues, Jack could entertain people for hours. For example, restaurant waitstaff were often at the center (not the brunt) of his humor. He had an amazing capacity to take common words or actions and make them quite comical. He'd have our friends in stitches. I reminded him often I married him primarily for his ability to make me laugh, and secondarily, of course, for his willingness to do the laundry and dishes.

A friend at his memorial service said exceptionally brilliant people see and feel the world in remarkably different ways than the rest of us. As a result, sometimes they fit in somewhere in the world, but mostly they don't. Sometimes they don't connect well with others because they feel things for which there is no description, so they just bury their emotions away to survive. In the end, among other physical, spiritual, and mental complexities, it was also this different perspective on life that contributed to Jack's difficulties. I came to understand, in retrospect, we had probably lived much of our lives with Jack on the cusp of life and of death. But that had become the norm for us. Possibly many people with mental health issues live on the edge, because every day can be a struggle. As a society, we just don't acknowledge nonconformity and mental distress as a natural part of living. People must live under societal norms that dictate they conform to the rest of the herd for fear of being labeled strange or, even worse, mentally compromised. So many people with mental and emotional struggles feel marginalized and isolated from the herd because they just can't conform to the norm. Social isolation can be further complicated by the fear they will be "found out" or even "thrown away" by society. Seeking treatment is the admission something is wrong, that you don't belong. As a society, we reinforce the idea with poorly funded mental health programs, the social stigma of mental illness, and, tragically, religious leaders who preach that sinful behaviors lead to mental health conditions or possessions and death of the soul.

A difficult childhood contributed to Jack's feelings of alienation in the world. He claimed he realized how important a loving and present family is for a child. However, through the years, he denied his upbringing in a fractured and distant family may have affected his coping skills or even his ability to love others. He seemed to always live on the outskirts of life and love like a satellite revolving around the Earth, desperately searching for signals but fearful he might find something. Because of this, he didn't develop critical pieces of himself that would have allowed him to feel whole as a human.

Sadly, in the end, it was simply time he wanted. He wanted back all the time he felt he had "wasted" in the wanting and wandering.

Additionally, it was curious how Jack perceived time. The idea of time had been a constant theme in our lives together. I was always asking for his time, whether for me or our boys.

He had read all of Stephen Hawking's works as well as other writings by great scientists. He understood time in a way most of us don't conceive. I tried to tell him early in our relationship time is not "of the essence" but *is* essence. Without investing in what is important to you in life, then time is a character in a book you can't write. It's the character who disappears the moment you see his face. If you aren't present and engaged, you miss it.

His early concepts of time were much different. He was *pressed for time*; he felt there was *no time like the present.* Later, time was like gold. He knew he'd be a rich man if he could just get it back again, but he couldn't. Time had escaped him like sand between open fingers.

Regardless, my time with him at the end became the most beautiful tragedy of my life. As I look back on the last three years of his life, it was my time he longed for, time to go back and do it all again. He needed time to reclaim memories, create pet names, snuggle; time to blow out candles and cheer at his sons' ballgames. He coveted the memories he missed along the way of carving pumpkins at Halloween and building gingerbread houses for Christmas. He wanted to hear little boys' voices in the morning as they bantered in the bathroom, to feel the gentle touch or the warm breath of a loved one beside him in bed. He wanted his time back—some, if not all. He wanted to experience the things that are birthed in each moment when we are present and engaged. Time became his enemy in the end—a noble adversary in the battle of life.

In the final days, he would say I told so many stories about daily life with the boys for which he had no points of reference. As we grow older and our children grow and thrive out in the world on their own, those stories mean so much more. He claimed he had none. In his mind, he had few stories, he had few memories, and he had few connections in the world. He had spent his time racing to be the best, the smartest, the wealthiest—or was he running from impending doom? He was good at obtaining what he valued early on in life, what so many men are conditioned to value: success, money, and recognition. We all want to be relevant to someone. Without taking the time to build moments and relationships, though, we have no memories to get us through tough times. Without memories, we don't feel relevant. Time makes memories, good and bad, but they irrevocably change who you are and how you are connected to others. I vividly remember Jack's panic-stricken eyes as he described the emptiness, fear, and loneliness his memories left him with in the quiet, hollow moments before he fell asleep every night. It was unsettling even for me.

In the end, he clearly announced it was time for him to go. It was time for him to start over in another life. His time was up. He was confident this was what he wanted and needed. He knew deep down he had another chance to begin again, but he was confident without resources, mentally, physically, and spiritually, it wouldn't be in this lifetime. There was no way to convince him of anything different.

Caregivers can get lost in the struggle. I was so lost some days I couldn't recall when I'd become the caregiver, when my children had become caregivers. When did we cross over into being a safety net for a man with debilitating mental illness? And through it all we struggled with our own "enough-ness", and whether we were sufficient to carry that burden. The slow churning of time is subtle and insidious. We lost ourselves without realizing it. After the clearing of the rubble, I found I had lost my identity. The cleanup has been hard but critical to my recovery.

Our boys and I have since moved on. In the aftermath, time and memories were both friends and foes. Early on, sometimes they were archenemies stealing away sleep, joy, and sanity, and then later, sometimes they were coveted and familiar friends bearing cherished glimpses of years of bittersweet strife.

Love without connection is like a seed fallen onto jagged rocks instead of fertile earth. Without the right resources, that seed cannot grow and thrive.

I hope you find resources in this book to help you push through one more day, week, month, or year. I hope you'll gain the strength and tools to face the worst you can imagine and push through, to rise up like a phoenix from the ashes, and recover a stronger, happier, kinder you.

1

THE BEGINNING OF THE END

THE WEATHER GREW COLD and unfriendly. Reflecting on that winter, I can't say whether it was really less friendly or if it was just the condition of our lives at the time. While life felt frozen in time some days, it wasn't. I was oblivious to what was to come, but felt paralyzed by the condition of my life at the time.

I returned from a morning visit with a good friend one day and found my husband, Jack, sitting at the dining room table, writing. He looked down, ears flushed, at the paper beneath his wrist and covered it casually, as if the teacher had caught him writing a love letter in class. I asked him what he was writing. It was in the form of a letter and seemed longer than anything I'd seen him write in the last few months.

"Help me," he pleaded.

"What are you working on? I'll try."

I scooted a dining room chair close beside him. Experiencing a moment of excitement, I thought maybe he was working on his résumé or even an employment application.

"Not this." As he peered down at the now-rumpled pages beneath his hand, he said, "I want you to help me leave."

I couldn't quite process what he was asking. "Are you leaving us?" I asked.

"No, not in that sense," he said, becoming agitated. "I'm tired. I'm ready to move on. I need a plan to leave this place. Please help me."

Though his words were ambiguous, I began to read between the lines.

I looked deep into his determined, smoky blue eyes, which had grown tired and frail. The lines on his face seemed to have deepened into canyons. We all get lines in our face over time. To me, they represent the years of knowledge we gain, laughter we experience, and years we spend together with those we love. I remember admiring the wizened faces of ancient papa-sans sitting on the sides of streets when I lived in Okinawa as a child. They contained so much joy and wisdom. These weren't the same kind of wrinkles. As Jack's health deteriorated, the wrinkles carved deeper furrows into his face, which made him appear more serious and burdened than usual.

He choked out a whisper. "You have to help me leave," he said. "I am done. There is nothing left for me here. You and the boys will be fine. I'm a burden on the family and the finances."

He retreated into a familiar, logical state of mind. He used it when he wanted to convince me of something I didn't agree with. This time was different though. His normally elaborate and complex language deteriorated into awkward sentences that were choppy and simplistic. He wasn't convincing at all.

He avoided eye contact, his posture oddly slumped toward the paper. What he said and his body language were wildly incongruent. It finally occurred to me he was giving up, and he was trying to do it in his typically "rational," unemotional manner.

A nauseating silence fell. The anger welled inside me. How could a man who loved me ask such a thing?

The heel of my hand slammed to the table, startling us both. "*No!* Stop this!" I hissed through clenched teeth. "I can't! I won't! Now you've asked too much!"

A sleeping volcano threatened to come alive. The pressure bubbled up from my whole being and relieved itself through a great gust of steam. Honestly, I thought by this stage of my life I had evolved to quite a different place spiritually than the one I'd started in as a child, yet my deep Southern Baptist upbringing ignited panic and judgment of his wishes to a degree that surprised me.

Regaining my composure, I called on help—help from deep inside of me. The kind of help you call on in a crisis; God, angels. Prayers of desperation filled my soul.

I resorted to blunt, simple sentences as if I were speaking to a child or sending out commands like a drill sergeant. I loathed speaking to him like that but, as his mental health had deteriorated, it became my response to his childlike behaviors. I didn't like it. I was in survival-mode.

I took a deep breath. I reminded myself I was tired from the many months of his deteriorating health, and his intense anxiety and panic in recent weeks.

I ignored his request.

Just like that. I ignored it.

I redirected the conversation.

The policy in our household for my children was a simple one: "Respect all living things at all times." I felt I was violating my own rule now. Many days I felt my own integrity was compromised. Many days I didn't like myself when I was with Jack. As much as I wanted to be patient and kind, somehow the long-standing patience I had been known for was eroding. I had become a stranger to myself.

I sent out more commands. "So, I think you should lie down. You're exhausted. I'm exhausted. No more talk like this. You don't mean it," I said it quickly and abruptly, so he couldn't interrupt.

I realized the volume of my voice had escalated and my posture had become defensive. I softened.

"Listen, I really have to do some work today. It will be okay." I was trying to muster an encouraging, soft voice while my insides were screaming.

I sunk back into reassuring him as I did almost every day. I hoped to move him past a position of defeat and into a more optimistic mood we could actually work with.

"Go lie down and we'll take a walk in a couple of hours. I promise." I said. "I promise."

I knew it wasn't the most respectful behavior to ignore his request but, as a survival technique, I had to pretend it wasn't there, out in the open. Because, on his worst days, I struggled to find time to work.

He was currently unemployed and my income was the only one keeping us afloat.

Jack always made a much higher income than I had. Our role reversal was hard on him, as a man and as a husband and father. After several months of him being unemployed, I realized this wasn't a temporary condition.

The previous year, I transitioned out of a university setting and found my stride running a business and consulting on international public health programs. I had embraced teaching. The proverbial "light going on" for students thrilled my soul. However, I could make more money to support the family as a consultant and business owner with all that was going on at home. I was happy with my decision. I felt much more productive, both academically and financially, as an independent contractor.

I rose from the dining table slowly. I felt as if a fog had dropped down over my ears. Jack mumbled his desires over and over. His words seemed so far away. As his begging became more desperate, I feared the escalation again. I became louder and more determined than before. I just couldn't—wouldn't—do this now.

The protector in me wanted to take care of him, to fix it. The exhausted guardian of my sanity decided to ignore the issue for the moment.

"It will all be okay." I said. "You're just tired. Please go lie down. I'll be done in a while and we can go for a walk."

I carefully gauged my words. Experience taught me to redirect rogue conversations quickly or they could decline to the point of Jack's emotions cycling in and out of unmanageable distress.

Deflated and dejected, he left the room.

I glanced down at his writing, which began, "To my loving wife, you have loved and cared for me for such a long time now. Thank you."

This was the opening to two pages of script. The existence of this letter seemed to cruelly mock my every effort to help him live. Without reading another word, I destroyed the letter as if it were the enemy.

To this day, I regret I didn't read it.

I moved from the room, shaken. My head pounded as if my heart had moved up inside it. My mind raced, looking for solutions.

I had already spent long hours waiting on hold, relentlessly trying to get Jack care somewhere—anywhere—as his mental stability degraded over the previous weeks. The wait times for hospitals, clinics, and private practices were ridiculously long. The soonest appointment I could secure was three weeks away. Given the rate at which his health was deteriorating, I didn't know how could we possibly endure this. I didn't know how I could *survive* without collapsing from full-body exhaustion.

I began to cry, the kind of crying you just can't afford to let out. It was trapped in my chest, gummy, like peanut butter, thick and unforgiving. A painful knot in my throat dropped down and embedded deeply in my heart.

Breathlessly, I tried to recover any composure I could muster to prevent the tears from falling. Tears are a way for the body to release stress, sadness, and other emotions that can harm it. Yet, there were times when I felt that if I released the raging river of tears, I might fall to the floor in a heap. Too much was at stake for me to risk becoming that vulnerable. I had to keep it together, like I had so many times before.

I retreated to my office to work, but I couldn't stay there. I eased into a hot shower, my one refuge where I could cry without repercussions. My chest heaved in pain. My heart hurt for him. It hurt for our kids and for the future. I felt hope slipping away.

The drama exasperated me. It was challenging enough to manage the deep depression and grief Jack experienced daily, but his emotions were complicated by panic and anxiety over what, to me, seemed like simple things. He experienced physical pain that prevented him from doing typical activities. The pain manifested intermittently at first but then seemed to grow like a malignant tumor every day. The number of fatal conditions and diseases he thought he had increased exponentially. Yet, modern medicine couldn't find anything physically wrong with him. For the twenty years I had known Jack, he didn't even take aspirin, and yet, here we were with ever-evolving stages of disease.

I wondered why he avoided doctors and medications through the years, but now I could only suspect he was concerned he'd be admitted to a psychiatric hospital and never released.

Now, for whatever reason, he was in a position of crisis. While I sympathized, I gazed upon his face every day wondering what had happened to the man I married.

Jack had morphed into someone almost unrecognizable. A deep-rooted, insidious, and consuming fear permeated his every word and action. The strong, confident jawline I'd admired so much had sunk back into his neck, and deep lines of worry had overtaken his face. His ocean-blue eyes had become steely gray and flat. Complicated by underlying depression, his anxiety had come out with a fury he couldn't suppress. Now he was unemployed and fragile, and his fear of failure intimidated his will to live.

He became terrified of failure, being alone, and being exposed as a fraud. Soon it became a fear of losing the love of his family, which he had squandered through the years. He felt too vulnerable, too exposed. He felt too intensely and too deeply to choose to live.

I dropped to my knees in the shower and curled up on the floor as if I were retreating into a chrysalis. I needed nourishment. I needed help.

After a liberating, cathartic cry, I felt I could face my life again, at least for now. With eyes swollen and burning, I climbed out of the shower, dressed, and sat down at the computer in my office to work.

Before long, I heard our two dogs barking in the house, startled into vigilance. What drew my attention first was simply that they were *in* the house. Though it was still chilly, they had been outside earlier, enjoying an unusually bright day. The erratic barking suggested there might be a postman at the door or someone reading the utility meter in the yard... but again, I wondered, why were the dogs in the house?

I listened to the intensity of the barks escalate for a few moments, but I kept working. Each day I squeezed out all the precious time I could to work before the door opened and another interruption ensued.

I tried to focus and allow the intrusion to resolve on its own. Within a few moments, a hush fell over the house. I believed the source of their irritation gone. Sighing with relief, I paused to recollect the ideas that had floated out of my brain.

After a short reprieve, more barking drew my attention again to the activity of the house. I opened the door to my office and noted the groan of door hinges installed in the 1920s. It seemed everything was irritable, even the house itself. When we'd first met the house, I had fallen in love with the gentle archways and the character it boasted. It seemed like the house had been loved through the generations. I felt I could hear the laughter of families in the old house, though it was just in my head. Quite possibly, it was laughter in our own family I so desperately needed.

Sometime in the past few years, Jack stopped laughing. He had the wittiest sense of humor of anyone I knew. He could bring an entire room to the point of hysteria with his comedic ranting. But through the years, his growing and relentless fear doused his laugh.

Jack resented the house from the beginning. I'm not sure why, but it was a source of irritation for him. Maybe it was because it was old and he felt there was always something to fix. Or maybe he also heard the laughing and it was a painful reminder of what he had lost, both as a child and in our own family, which he had hoped would repair him.

I left my office. As I moved through the house, I inspected each room, until I reached the den, where the barks originated. I glanced at both of the dogs as I hurried by in my bare feet but just gave them the usual "hush" and continued to dart through the house. They quieted for a moment, but only long enough for me to leave the room.

To check if Jack had been disturbed, I cracked open the door of the room Jack had retreated to. He wasn't there.

As the dogs' barks echoed, I began to move through the house faster. Something was awry. There was a heaviness to the air, and a feeling of dread overtook me.

Was he in the bathroom? The kitchen?

A rapid increase in my heart rate and a blanket of chills told me instinctively something was wrong.

I imagine the sense I had is akin to what people who volunteer for search-and-rescue missions experience. I knew whatever situation I found could not possibly turn out well. A feeling of impending doom resonated throughout the nooks and shadows of the house.

As I passed through the dining room, the table where Jack and I had been sitting just an hour earlier was neat and tidy. I noticed new papers on the table. I hadn't a clue where they had come from or why they were there, but I didn't stop to investigate. I just assumed Jack was organizing all the bills, receipts, and other documents in his usual fashion.

The clicking of the dogs' nails on the large windowpanes and their agitated bellows refocused my attention. I walked back to the den to calm them and let them out.

What did they see?

I looked over their wagging tails and lunging bodies to see something moving in the woods outside. I thought the next-door neighbors' stout, black, charismatic Lab mutt, Max, may have once again wriggled through a hole in our fence.

The year before, a fallen tree gouged a hole in the large fence surrounding our property. The trees and brush were thick enough it was difficult to reach it for repairs. Our aging, mostly lazy border collies rarely ventured from the comfort of the back porch, so it had never been fixed. Now and then a roaming wild animal— or Max—would make its way into the backyard.

As I approached the back door, I noticed it was ajar. Leaving the house with bare feet and wet hair, I walked toward the edge of the woods but could barely make out the figure. When I moved closer, I realized it was human.

Cautiously, I called out, "Hello?"

I called three times, increasing in volume with each call. Finally, the figure turned. As he looked at me, I saw an apologetic expression of true desperation through barren winter trees. I had the surreal experience of feeling within the same moment I knew this man and yet I didn't. My brain couldn't comprehend the magnitude of what I thought I saw. Time stood still.

Soldiers returning from war describe events that occurred in just a matter of seconds in such great detail it's as if the events lingered on endlessly. In that instant, seconds seemed to expand into unmeasurable units. The air was crushing, thick and unforgiving. I couldn't breathe.

The realization Jack had a gun in his hand propelled me into panic. Adrenaline flooded my body and my heart exploded in a rhythm audible inside my head. A guttural and primal noise permeated the air. I screamed, but it was as if the voice were not my own. As I recall that moment, I remember that scream more vividly than most other things. I belted out Jack's name as if he were in the path of an oncoming and out-of-control vehicle.

I screamed again, "Jack, *come here*! *Now!* Drop the gun and come here!" I startled even myself. It wasn't my voice or one I had ever heard come from my body. It was a booming, authoritative voice from nowhere... or from everywhere. My heart pounded so loudly I could barely think.

2

REFLECTIONS ON THE PAST

MY FAMILY'S ROOTS ARE IN Southeastern Oklahoma, near the Choctaw Nation in Broken Bow. Most of my family, on both sides, lived there, but my mother and father felt the only way out of poverty was for him to enlist with the United States Air Force. I have come to greatly appreciate their decision to leave the area, regardless of its amazing beauty and crystal-clear lake. For them, with little industry and few jobs, Broken Bow was a sentence of lifelong poverty. The military offered the resources we needed to become the family we are today. This sense of family and love kept us together as we moved from airbase to airbase.

My mother would say, "Home is where you are, not where you've been." Conditioned with that thought as a child, I was sad initially when we moved from place to place but never felt insecure. The military provided a way out of poverty and a way into cultural experiences.

I was born in California and lived in Oklahoma for a short while, but my earliest memories are from when we were stationed at Kadena Air Base in Okinawa. My brother and I were very young. It was a culture shock to all of us at first, but my brother, Sam, and I were young enough to adapt quickly. I was six and he was almost two. When we first arrived, there was no housing available on the airbase, so we lived off the base among Okinawan families who quickly became our friends.

I have wonderful memories from there. I remember visiting the Japanese fish markets and the Buddhist temple with my friends and their parents. I have vivid memories of staying with Japanese Girl Scouts in exchange programs. None of us spoke the other's language, but it didn't seem to matter. We would play hide-and-seek among the tombs in the Okinawan cemetery on warm, balmy Saturdays. We would jump up on the gray, sun-bleached stone walls lining the houses off base and bask in the sun while we shared a piece of sugarcane from the field down the road. As an enlisted military kid, I remember knowing no discrimination or racial bias. We were just happy to have friends.

Regardless of these and many other happy memories, my home was where the family was, and the places we left quickly became only distant memories. I grew up seeing how love can ground a family, despite its changing location. My mother was deeply involved in giving us time and attention, creating memories and traditions. Fiercely protective, she was loving and sometimes generous to a fault. I also came to realize she was progressive in her parenting for the time period. And after learning about her turbulent childhood, complete with neglect and abuse, it's even more surprising she could muster the skills to be an exceptional parent.

My parents never denied us much of anything, though, as an adult, I experienced the stark realization we were very poor during my early childhood years. Thankfully, I never felt the weight poverty can have on families.

My size made it possible for me to wear my clothes year after year (my father called me a beanpole, affectionately, until middle school). My mother sewed strips of material to the bottom of my pants to lengthen them. My favorite pants became new, year-by-year, as my mother decorated them with different rickrack and lace, as was the fashion at the time. Trick-or-treating with homemade costumes sewn from scraps made me feel special, though apparently this was traumatic for Sam, who one year protested that "Batman is just not green!!"

Being enlisted military meant we just couldn't afford new clothes, new costumes, or the luxury of hair products. For example, she slathered mayonnaise on her head—and sometimes mine—to condition her naturally curly auburn hair. She wrapped it up in a towel and we went about our business for close to an hour looking like we had turbans tightly wrapped around our heads. For years in my young adulthood, I marinated in mayonnaise with a towel turban around my head and I felt smart —like I was somehow beating the system.

My mother ingrained in us the value of an education and virtues of religion. She told me an education would get you anything in life you needed, and God would give you direction and grace along the way. The military provided a very ecumenical church experience, opening my mind on rotating Sundays to the Episcopal, Methodist, Pentecostal, and Presbyterian faiths. I attended the Catholic service sometimes with my friend Jackie, whose family came from Puerto Rico. My love of God was deep. I look back and realize these diverse experiences with religion and spirituality actually set the stage for my open-minded beliefs (which are usually more liberal than those of the rest of my family) about race, culture, religion, and acceptance of others.

I felt supported and encouraged, and sometimes intense pressure to do my very best. But my childhood wasn't free from pain. My Pollyanna tendencies were checked at the state line during our annual visits to family in Oklahoma. Poverty in our extended family stretched far and deep. I remember visiting Aunt Alice, who sat in a rocking chair and spit "baccy" in a spittoon. My grandma on my mother's side, who was related to Aunt Alice, was half Choctaw, and my grandfather was a first-generation American from Ireland.

My dad's father died of cancer when I was in middle school. His mother died of either "consumption" or cancer—records weren't that explicit back then—when my father was only sixteen. As an adult, I realized how difficult that must have been when I lost my own mother at twenty-one.

We seldom visited family. I never imagined there was any particular reason. I just thought excursions around the world in the military kept us away. As I got older, I understood. I learned about awful secrets in the family. There was significant mental, physical, and sexual abuse—including for me when I was there. Years after my mother's death, I learned of the mistreatment and abuse she experienced as a little girl, which explained why it was necessary for her to keep distance between us and them.

My father had to grow up on his own, scrapping for himself mostly. He said after his mother died, his dad "just quit trying." My memories of my dad in the early years are few but dear. He was fun and goofy much of the time but he had a kind and gentle side as well. To my mother's dismay, he was the fun guy and she was the disciplinarian.

When I experienced excruciating headaches as a child, he held pressure on my head until I fell asleep. When I had a nightmare, he came into my room and provided an airtight rationale for letting go of the terror I felt. He convinced me despite my bad dreams, all was right with the world. As most young daughters of respectable fathers probably do at some point, I huddled with my five-year-old best friend, Jennie, in a mud puddle beneath the mimosa tree in our front yard making "pies" and claimed my dad as my boyfriend, stating I would marry him one day. I distinctly remember the flash of sun on her pretend aluminum foil braces as she emphatically lisped out, "Dads cannot be boyfriends!"

I was devastated for days.

Though he was called to duty much of the time, my father was loving and attentive when he was home. However, I realized later in life his absences impacted my personal relationships with men. I found through the years many of my female friends have had this same experience.

It makes sense now that I know how critically influential father-and-daughter relationships are to the development of healthy adult relationships with men. Growing up, I had what I thought to be a wonderful relationship with my father when he was home and available. However, his service to the military took him away often, so he had to leave most of the child rearing to my mother. Military moms are some of the strongest women in the world but still quite vulnerable. Military personnel are at risk in all aspects of their jobs. When he was gone, she had to be brave, and what we perceived at times to be controlling, to keep order in a family faced with uncertainty.

My father was sent on temporary duty for extended periods of time, sometimes with no idea about the danger he would encounter or when we would next see him. There were also gaps in regular military pay. I have memories of my mother, her voice whisper-strained so we couldn't hear, cupping her hand over the phone to ask another military mom if they had gotten paid that month. My mother had to run the household on a very tight budget. My father was gone often and she had to trust we would be able to eat some months.

My father relayed what he thought was a funny story about my mother hiding a bar of chocolate she bought at the commissary. He accidentally found the hidden Hershey bar fumbling in a drawer. She looked as if she had been caught with her hand in the cookie jar. I never thought this was a funny story. The poverty was tragic and the chiding seemed to humiliate her.

As I grew older and wiser, I deeply understood and respected her need for stability. I understood while she loved my father, she could not trust his or the military's support would always be there for her and her children. Out of this I learned I needed to be self-sufficient. There was always a chance I would need my own income and I took that very seriously.

My parents were the first on both sides of my family tree to go to college. The military afforded my parents that opportunity. They both graduated from college near Barksdale Airforce Base where we were stationed. At the time, my brother and I were in middle and high school, respectively. Given their circumstances and challenges, this was quite a feat for both of them. They completed college with honors. My mother became a teacher and my father an engineer, and we were so proud. We celebrated successes and grieved together in failures, illnesses, and personal family losses.

My mother lived a short life. We lost her to breast cancer when she was forty-one years old. She'd been diagnosed shortly after she received her master's degree in counseling. The cancer was brutal and aggressive. A champion of resolve, she was determined to win against her illness. Until her final days, she went to work, at the magnet school where she taught, attached to an oxygen tank. She loved teaching fifth grade. After she graduated with her master's, they hired her to be a counselor at the very school where she taught. Though she was already ill, she was eternally optimistic. What many people didn't see, however, is that many days she would cry from exhaustion and pain when she got home. She began losing weight and got so winded she would have to stop and rest every few feet.

We knew she was losing the fight. My father frantically searched for natural remedies and treatments, even ordering supplements from a Caribbean country. Western medicine failed us, so anything and everything was on the table. She was deeply spiritual and believed she would be healed. And because she did, we did too. Or at least we wanted to believe it more than anything in the world.

As desperation set in, she went to see a spiritual healer in a Pentecostal church. She had grown up Assembly of God and in her hour of need returned to her roots. Though he professed to be a Christian, the healer said her faith was not strong enough and that was why the cancer was winning. Throughout her remaining time on this earth, she thought her personal faith was substandard. It grieved me to watch how deeply this affected her. Eventually, it took over her psyche. The irony was her faith was strong enough to move mountains and compassionate enough to change lives.

Unfortunately, her experience planted a seed of doubt in my mind about formalized religion I couldn't ever shake. I understand now the power of belief, mind over matter, but it was the way his words killed her spirit that crushed me.

Knowing she was ill, I chose to marry much sooner than I should have. I wanted her to be at my wedding. I wanted her to see me happy. Though she opposed it, I married a boy from high school at the age of twenty. I had no business marrying at such a young age, but I felt my very foundation was leaving the world. The prospect of life without her shook and frightened me.

Her struggle was harsh and cruel. Every day on the way home from university, I stopped at Sonic to get her a double chocolate shake for calories.

She died the following year.

Her final night alive affects me to this day. Accepting she was close to death, my father invited all family members to visit her. Friends and family came and went. People we hadn't seen for years came to sit with her. Though married, I stayed with her each day and night, fearing the worst but, of course, praying for the best.

One evening, I came home from university to hear her wonderful, infectious laugh bellowing from her bedroom—one of those laughs that came up from her toes and exploded in the room. When she laughed, everyone followed even if they had no clue what was so funny. Before long, the room was in tears— happy tears.

Her friends from days past surrounded her, and my grandmother perched in her bed. Tears rolled down their faces, and they laughed until they could barely breathe. My mother always loved to laugh and was quite funny herself. All of my family appreciated humor, whether slapstick, juvenile, snarky, or otherwise. I remember so many times my mother laughed until she cried, barely able to speak. I hadn't heard that beautiful sound in months.

That evening, I remember thinking she was going to be fine. The oxygen line was off her face and lay beside her in bed. She had not been able to function without oxygen for months. I thought it must be a miracle. I hadn't seen her this happy in months and months. She was acting like the mother I had known before cancer had insidiously stepped in to control our lives. We had been waiting for the next shoe to drop for two years. The weight of the worry we had lived with lifted. Free from care that evening, I went to dinner with a friend and decided to go home to my new husband for a change.

She died that night.

She died deep in the wee hours, too deep for us to recognize it and bring her back. My grandmother slept beside her at the time. She awoke to my mother's last gasps for life and made sure we heard that story over and over. It was distressing to hear at the time, but I now think it was probably important for her own healing to verbalize it.

By the time I reached the hospital, my mother was gone. I walked into the room completely confused about her decline after what I'd seen the evening before. I felt like I had been turned inside out.

The pain I experienced in those moments is the only rival of the absolute evisceration I felt the day Jack died. It took years for me to forgive myself for not being there when she died. There are days I still struggle with my decision to leave that night, though rationally I know there was nothing I could have done to save her.

Since then, I've learned my mother's experience is fairly typical of the way we leave the earth when we die. Many professionals have noted when someone is ready to go on to the next stage, they often seem as if they are much better, much happier, at peace. A lesson I failed to recognize even later in my life, when I needed it most.

Years after her death, I found an old cassette tape she'd used as a student in college. She'd read aloud her study notes. It was how she studied best. I was lulled to sleep many nights in high school listening to her voice resonating through our small but warm house as she read her class notes aloud.

On one side of the casette, she read notes from an undergraduate botany course. On the other side, she read notes from a graduate course for her master's degree, Abnormal Child Psychology. The difference in my mother's voice from one side of the audiotape to the next was astounding. Her use of language and her accent transformed dramatically, as, assuredly, my mother herself had.

I hardly remember my mother having a Southern accent, but she read those botany notes with such a strong drawl it made me chuckle. At first, I didn't believe it was her. On the reverse side, she read like a scholar, with perfect diction and in a familiar professional voice. I remember that voice the most. Outside of the occasional country saying, like "Well, that beats all I've ever stepped in," she spoke like an academic. I realized the power of education the instant I heard her voice transform. My parents reached their goal of breaking the cycle of poverty through education. I believe their achievement will save us for generations to come.

I grieved losing her for years, but it wasn't until I had my first baby I felt her absence most intensely. David was born four years after her death and I had no one to show me the way. I dreamed about her holding David, playing with him on the shag carpet, and sitting in the first row, proud eyes connecting with him at his kindergarten graduation. My marriage to David's father ended badly after 8 years. My mother's voice gently saying, "I told you that you both were too young" rang in my head for years afterward.

* * *

Jack's family held education in the highest regard. His family had a long history of children attending the best colleges in the nation and abroad. Education was not so much an achievement as an expectation. Because of their drive for learning, his family was wealthy relative to mine, owning large businesses and engaged in professional careers as far back as one could research. Jack was not only extremely intelligent by academic standards, but he was also "book and world" educated, extending his knowledge beyond that of most people in society.

What I didn't know was that his affinity for words and reading, his drive for excellence and hard work, and his appreciation for precision and detail, were excessive. I had no reference for his world when we met. Though always very kind to me, his family seemed fragmented and at times antagonistic and competitive with one another. The battles of wits that raged between them on holiday visits occasionally left me feeling shell-shocked.

Jack's biological father, Barry, was absent most of his life. When he was twenty-seven, Jack sought out a relationship with him. He asked his grandmother where he could find his father. Jack often recalled memories of writing lyrics and music on the guitar about his father when he was young. He longed to know him but feared rejection and held reservations about how it would affect his mother. When he finally met him, he began a meaningful "friendship" with him—"but that's all," Jack would say.

Barry became a significant part of our lives. He was kind but intense. He too hailed from a family that had done well for themselves. He had been a banker in Dallas, back when bankers did quite well. Tales of backroom gambling and high-stakes risk-taking were a part of his legacy. He was a connoisseur of fine wines and smooth whiskey. He loved to have parties and "get-togethers" with friends. He lived to impress, but not in a flashy way. He enjoyed the finer things in life, but as an older man, he never seemed selfish. He was quite generous with gifts, money, and support for his family when needed. Meeting Barry, I understood a lot about Jack. Although Jack didn't grow up with him, the apple doesn't fall far from the tree. Jack had so many of his mannerisms and behaviors it was surreal sometimes. Barry was a take-no-prisoners kind of guy when it came to business. He had a commanding presence and an uproarious laugh that startled everyone in the room. Barry had two other sons, who were quite surprised to learn they had an older half-brother. I'm sure it was hard on both of them.

Mere teens when they met, Jack's mother, Diane, and Barry found themselves expecting after a brief intimate encounter one summer. They married, but I suspect it was mostly out of obligation. They were both so very young and ill-prepared to take care of each other, much less a newborn baby. Neither of them was prepared to be a parent.

To complicate things, Jack's mother, Diane, suffered with her own significant depression after Jack was born. She was hospitalized. Her pregnancy was distressing and probably worsened her condition.

Another family member told me Jack's grandmother stepped in to care for him while Barry worked and Diane was in the hospital. She also cared for him for many years off and on thereafter.

Though they were mostly well-educated and accomplished, many of Jack's family members suffered from disorders, including bipolar, schizophrenia, depression, and other conditions. Long medical histories of hospitalizations and medical management peppered the genetic line on both sides of Jack's family tree.

Diane and Barry remained married a brief three years, long enough to add another baby, Lucy, to their list of responsibilities. Soon, divorce ensued, and Diane got custody of Jack and his young sister, with limited rights for Barry. Contrary to Diane's recall, Barry shared stories of attempted visits and money he sent. He desperately wanted Jack to know he was wanted and loved. Regardless of the truth, for Jack it came too late in the course of his life.

Jack's stepfather, Hal, also a brilliant mind, impressed upon Jack the value of reading and learning. He embraced the idea education and "smarts" will get you most things in life. Jack took this to heart and always tried to impress him. Hal was Jack's father figure though they seemed to have a laissez-faire type relationship. They engaged intellectually but never interfered with each other's lives.

Jack probably related most to Hal. Hal was his role model. They both approached relationships mostly with logic. Hal was kind but could be perceived as cold and unfeeling because of the practical way he approached life. Of Jack's family, I found Hal the easiest to understand. Nothing was hidden with him. Like it or not, you knew exactly where you stood with him.

I learned much about life from Jack's family. They warmly accepted me and my son into the fold, but I never quite comprehended the family dynamics with which he grew up.

Jack was unpredictable and a free spirit. His mother would share stories about his childhood and how difficult he was to manage. He was bright and curious and often conjured up trouble, so much trouble he spent two years of high school living in a home for troubled boys. His grandfather, a juvenile judge, established the home. Jack's exasperated mother placed him there (not the court system) but to his detriment, he learned much from suite mates who were there as a result of prior convictions.

Jack also learned discipline. He felt he personally benefitted from a strict schedule and the discipline the home enforced.

At the home, Jack also met a mentor, Dan, who took him under wing. Dan was a young, single veterinarian who volunteered to spend time with the boys, hoping to make an impact. He taught Jack important lessons about life he'd missed growing up. Dan was kind but also a stern disciplinarian. Jack described Dan as the only person who believed in him, other than his grandmother. While Dan wasn't physically demonstrative, he invested in Jack. Jack needed that investment.

Jack was definitely a risk taker, but only in matters of the mind, it seemed, never the heart. Early in our relationship, I assumed approaching relationships more logically was a reflection of how advanced education was expressed in families, yet it seemed adversarial and unloving at times. I felt unsophisticated and academically clumsy around his family. I drilled myself on vocabulary and which utensil to use for which course before going to his grandmother's house.

At times, I felt his family was oddly close, yet there seemed to be something sorely missing between them. Over time, Jack shared memories of ruined holidays and family rifts, but he relished the argumentative bantering that occurred when they got together. It was what he knew. His knowledge of words and language had been honed over the years, initially to protect himself from his own family and then to "win" in the world. It was so very foreign to me.

Stories about Jack as a child told by his family left me feeling like he had been a boy crying out for help from as young as the age of five, rather than a "problem child." I thought deeply about whether I was just too sensitive, because he seemed unfazed. They seemed to delight in his failures. It was surreal for me to listen to the pleasure they took in discussing what a rabble-rouser he was, always in trouble.

He would rarely share with me, but when he did, he told stories of what I perceived as emotional and physical neglect, and situations when he was left to fend for himself from a very young age. My impression was he was never really held or adored, comforted or nurtured. He seemed to feel "in the way" all of his life. In rare moments, he would share about his family dynamics. "They always chose someone or something else. They never chose me," he would say in a moment of vulnerability. He acted as if it didn't matter.

I still feel I know little about the depths of his family's condition because everyone has different recollections, but the effects of his upbringing challenged our own relationship.

Jack didn't dwell long on family stories. They were packed in tight inside him, like the rubber bands inside a golf ball. I felt like if I tapped into it at all and unleashed it, what was inside could hurt everyone in the room.

I took great caution whenever I asked him to open a door into his world. On occasion, when a door opened, he would interrupt his memory, slam it abruptly, and snarl, "Yeah, well, I was over that a long time ago. It doesn't affect me anymore." He would boast he was very adept at taking care of himself and referenced being left alone for sometimes days at a time to take care of his younger sister.

A child should never be expected to just survive. In our society, so many children are left to fend for themselves. This doesn't leave external bruises or scars, but the internal scars don't heal easily. Studies show neglect causes children to withdraw into themselves, leaving them with feelings of low self-esteem, inadequacy, and self-hatred. To survive, many of them take on a façade opposite their self-image. Some children overcompensate for the lack of confidence by becoming overconfident and engaging in risky behavior.

Jack was exactly that, overconfident and a risk taker. He desperately reached out for attention. As a child he caused trouble because some days that was the only way he could get attention. He would acknowledge he knew if he caused a reaction in his mother, it was better than no attention at all. He perceived his childhood environment to be, at best, uninviting.

* * *

Why was I attracted to Jack, then, particularly since I knew what a loving relationship should look like? Why was he attracted to me?

I have come to believe we each approach life in the best way we know how, given the resources we have at the time. We choose relationships to meet our basic unmet needs. Deep within we seek out people whom we can comfortably navigate. However, we also seek out people who harbor resources we don't have in our toolbox. I believe today I was comfortable with Jack's "absence" in our relationship because I associated relationship absence with the value of work. My father's work kept him away, but it was also our only source of support.

I valued education and culture because of what my mother taught me and my experiences as a military kid. I had no idea how to obtain those resources for myself. I longed to further the evolution my parents began, from our family's roots toward a better life for generations to come, but I lacked the self-confidence to move forward. Plus, I had neither the fiscal resources nor the knowledge to get there. I needed Jack's drive for knowledge, understanding of the world, ability to navigate it, and confidence to do it.

He needed my resources. He needed the love and trust of a devoted, unconditional family. He needed to be chosen for who he was and what he offered to the world.

3

WHAT WAS US

REFLECTING ON THE STORY that was us, we were definitely an enigma as a couple. We exemplified the idea "opposites attract," and throughout our twenty years together we became polarized in such a way we rarely encroached on each other's world. Some days were uplifting and beautiful—and some very destructive. I loved him and I believe he loved me. I told him through the years I loved him in a way that I didn't understand, but it would be easier if we each lived on our own side of a duplex. Meaning, of course, I couldn't live with the man, nor could I live without him.

It seems like a lifetime ago I met Jack. *A Brief History of Time* by Stephen Hawking in hand, he read quietly and intently in the hospital auditorium awaiting a seminar. His silhouette against the lit stage stood out against the shadow of the seating area. An all-consuming book rendered him oblivious to his surroundings. My voice startled him and he looked above his John Lennon–style glasses. I remember thinking—counter to my first impressions of him—he was geekishly attractive.

We worked at the same hospital, in the same department. He was relatively new and when he arrived, chip on his shoulder, I wasn't impressed. However, there was something about him... an intrigue. I wondered whether I was drawn to the proverbial "bad boy" attitude. I sure didn't need that in my life! Now, in the auditorium, I realized that he wasn't the bad-boy type at all. He was more of an intellectual, a geek on steroids. But it didn't really matter; I didn't have the time for a relationship.

Curious, though, I inquired about his book and we began a conversation I never imagined would result in marriage. At the time, I was put off by his poor interpersonal skills. He was abrupt and matter-of-fact, seemingly impatient with my inquiry. He was bright and well-read but carried an air about him that was elusive and sometimes abrasive. In a condescending voice, he stated I should have read Hawking's book. Interestingly, what felt like an insult made me think about my environment and childhood development. Why hadn't I read such books? It felt rude at the time, but he always had the capacity to make me think about the world in a different way. Yes, he was arrogant and intolerable at times, but it piqued my interest to be challenged by subjects about which I knew so little.

Not long after we met that day, Jack left a note under the door of my office at the hospital. He asked if he could take me to brunch after playing a game of basketball. Stemming from the conversation in the auditorium, he knew I played point guard in high school and challenged me to a game.

Now a single mom, trying to keep it all together, I had so little time with David. It had been almost six months since I'd separated from David's dad. I worked long hours. At the time, his father was barely present. We were both so young, too young—as emphasized by my mother—when we married, and ultimately found we had different interests and life goals; we were very different people. The stress of my mother's death, our financial worries, and our being ill equipped for marriage in general led to discontent in the relationship. When life got too difficult after David's birth, I decided to leave. But regardless of the relationship between his dad and me, we loved David.

I asked myself over and over... did I really want to be in a relationship again? Should I accept the invitation and see why I was so intrigued by Jack? Or just follow my instincts and politely decline like I had so many times in the "meat market" hospital environment?

I was wary, but curious, so I accepted. I insisted we go Dutch at brunch, because I wanted to send him a clear signal I wasn't a pushover and I could take care of myself. We had a wonderful time. It was easy to talk with him, unlike previous dates—lunch with the pediatric cardiologist who was strangely obsessed with his body, or the Renaissance festival with the pulmonologist who felt compelled to scoff at my pronunciation of Celtic.

This time it felt real. It felt natural. And for a few hours, I felt like I was engaging in interesting and important conversations. He was bright, funny, and considerate.

Now, as I look back, I understand we each held resources for which the other longed. Like two opposing but interconnecting circuits, it all fit together so easily. Our views were like oil and water when it came to many issues, but the resistance was natural and cooperative. We challenged each other in a way that created a tension that pulled us together rather than apart. And though I was occasionally annoyed by it, I found myself drawn into his world. We began to go to events with mutual friends and eventually with just one another.

The relationship was platonic for quite some time. We both had limited time to give to dating. When we met, I had a developing career in medical staff development and a young son who needed my attention and care. He was the absolute center of my world. As a single mother with the responsibility of raising a son, I was cautious about moving into a relationship again.

Jack approached his career with great dedication and worked many hours. I saw him as our schedules permitted, and I was fine with that. I was busy with David and work. Eventually we began prioritizing our time together. Because of his schedule, I mostly saw him in the late evenings as he came off a twelve-hour shift in the hospital. A couple of evenings a month, he arrived after David was asleep. I'd cook something to eat and then we'd sit on the floor talking until the wee hours of the morning as he massaged pressure points on my feet. Sometimes he'd slip in at eleven p.m., an hour before he went to work on the night shift. He worked two jobs and often worked double shifts. I admired his work ethic. In most of my previous relationships, I had been the sole breadwinner in the relationship, barely making ends meet. I appreciated he valued hard work and maintaining his income, so I wasn't concerned about how little time we spent with one another.

When we did spend time together, he made me laugh. He was remarkably funny. He was a gentleman and seemed respectful of others. There were times when I questioned his judgment, and if I had been worldlier, I guess I would have recognized there was something odd about his personality. Many times, when we were out in public or at an event with David, he would disappear for uncomfortable lengths of time without notice. Sometimes an hour or two would go by with no word about where he was. I would become worried and go searching for him. When I was on the brink of calling the police or finding security, he would show up with a story about helping a stranded traveler in the parking lot or attending to a work issue on the phone. Regardless, I felt it was insensitive and thoughtless of him not to consider he might be worrying us. Behaviors like these were nagging red flags of things to come.

Inherent to his personality was skepticism of conventional thought. Seldom did he agree with popular ideas or succumb to popular culture. He would say he didn't celebrate Valentine's Day because it was a commercial holiday. If he wanted to buy me flowers, he could buy them any day of the week. (Of course, that would be if he actually thought of buying flowers now and then— but he didn't.)

He also said not to expect he return an "I love you" because he didn't want the phrase to be a reflexive, meaningless response to my emotion. I bought into this thought early on because it made sense I should not rely on someone telling me he loved me —how needy! Actions speak louder than words, I thought. Unfortunately, I realized late in the relationship those beliefs were not true. I did need to be told I was loved. My father declared after my mother's death he would say, "I love you" to his kids at every opportunity because you never know when you'll lose the chance. We all agreed with him.

Over the course of time, brainwashed, I became harder and more cynical myself. I bought into Jack's ideas because I have a little bit of deep cynicism and suspicion of conspiracy at the core of my being, too. He spoke with such authority and confidence I believed most of what he said.

Before I knew it, I was in. I was all-in. And I believe Jack was in with all he had to give, although, because of his childhood, "all-in" meant something very different to him. "All-in" to me was a way of life. It was a full commitment to the relationship. But my definition of "all-in" was in a language he didn't understand. He told me once no one had everbeen all-in for him without strings attached, so he was wary of the commitment. He felt he always needed a backup plan or a back door—a way out—to feel comfortable.

Despite my nagging concerns, we married on the evening of a cold Thanksgiving Day. We intended to make things more convenient for visiting family members, but I think by and large, it turned out to be an inconvenience to everyone. We held a small wedding at his house. The house was immense but completely unfurnished, except with futons and a television. It was cold much of the time in the winter. While it worked well for a wedding venue, it was a metaphor for how he functioned in the world: larger than life on the outside, but empty on the inside.

At the time, I remember thinking this was just bachelor behavior and I could change things, but I was remarkably wrong. During the year we spent living in this house, he was frustratingly spartan and restrictive with finances. Despite my ongoing protests, the house remained unfurnished and cold.

David was a happy boy, but Jack was often disengaged when he was home. He carried on working long hours. He also traveled for his new job with a medical technology company. He trained physicians and medical personnel to use new equipment in hospitals around the country. As much as I begged him to slow down, there was a new imperative in his life: the burden of taking care of a family. It gave rise to a new level of busyness, and he had a justification for it.

About six months into the marriage, I was elated to find I was pregnant. We weren't necessarily trying to have a baby, but we weren't preventing it either. Jack treated nearly everything in his life like a game of Russian roulette. He never planned anything for fear of failure or disappointment. His tumultuous and unpredictable childhood ingrained in him he should avoid setting expectations. If he planned something and it failed, he could say, "Oh, I didn't intend for that to happen anyway."

So while he was fearful of having a child, he refused to use protection. If it happened by "accident," then he couldn't be disappointed either way. It was a logic I understand now, given what I learned through the years, but I thought it was ridiculous at the time.

I was very ill during this pregnancy. I hadn't been sick one day when I was pregnant with David. From the beginning, I intuitively felt something was wrong, but I justified it by saying, "It must be a girl." Playing into wives' tales was a specialty of mine, the influence of humble family roots, uneducated and marked with Ozark mountain fables and beliefs. Or maybe it was a blend of American Indian lore with a staunch Southern Baptist upbringing. Regardless, I had many beliefs running around in my head.

What I do remember is the day I lost her. Jack had been out of town for several days. Actually, I had begun to feel better. After weeks of spot bleeding and being bedridden for several days, I thought the pregnancy was taking a turn for the better. I was sixteen weeks along.

That night, I had a remarkably powerful and vivid dream. A pretty but frail little girl of about seven came to me and reached out her hand. She had long brown hair and big hazel eyes. It was one of those dreams where you keep asking yourself if you're awake, and yet you know it's a dream.

I recognized her to be my daughter. Though she never said, I knew her name was Mila. I took her little hand in mine and noticed she looked very ill. Her eyes were dark and sad. She said, "I'm sorry, Mommy, but I have to leave you."

I jolted awake. A strong perfume wafted through the bedroom. I knew that perfume, and somehow, I knew it was my father's mother coming to take the baby with her. Though I felt very alone in the darkness, also I felt the calming presence of my grandmother—strangely, the one I didn't know. I wept tears of grief—grief I didn't understand.

David typically climbed into bed with me at some point in the night, but he wasn't there. Rattled, I rose and walked down the hall to check on him. He lay there sleeping so sweetly. I always found a renewed strength when I looked at him. I knew when he was born he was an old soul. Tears flowing, I was so grateful for the beautiful little human he was and the amazing man I knew he would be. It was in that moment I knew I had to let the baby go.

Dreading the results, the next day I went in to see my doctor. Time expanded during the sonogram, as I lay, belly exposed, on the exam table. Relentless tension rose in the room after several minutes of silence and I began to cry. I knew. I knew what I had experienced was not just a dream but a confrontation with death. I had a history of prophetic dreams, and I knew.

The doctor pulled a tissue from a nearby cardboard box, and while laying it gently on my stomach, he said, "I'm sorry but you've lost your baby."

He exited the room, leaving me to cry on the table, feeling alone again. The tears streamed down my face uncontrollably. I wiped them like I was trying to conceal them but they kept coming. I sat up as a nurse entered the room to ask if I wanted a picture of my baby girl from the sonogram. I was shocked and angered and snapped back, "Why would I want a picture? She's gone."

I question that strong response to this day, but I think it stemmed from a place of anger, grief, and sorrow. I called Jack when I got home and he flew home the next day. Weeks of rationale for why it was "better to lose her than to have a baby with deformities" followed. It was Jack's way of justifying what had happened. It didn't help me. I would have loved her anyway, but he was probably right.

What it did to him was most troubling to me. It made him even more unsure of his ability to do anything right. He belabored the idea he'd never wanted children anyway and that he had never seen himself married, much less as a father. This was his way of protecting himself. Life is always messy but he wanted it to be perfect. If he was perfect, then life would be perfect, and no one could criticize him. He knew he couldn't bear imperfection in the health of a child and I think God knew that too.

By the next year, I was pregnant with Josh. While I understood there could be a repeat loss, I wanted another baby and a sibling for David, and Jack finally agreed. Unfortunately, Jack was very disengaged with this pregnancy, because he didn't want to be disappointed, I'm sure. He didn't want to feel like he'd failed me and David. He showed brief moments of excitement, especially when the baby moved or kicked, but ultimately disconnected from the experience. It caused deep sadness in me because I felt alone in the pregnancy sometimes. I so wanted to have a partner to share this precious baby with and it was already looking doubtful.

In the later days of the pregnancy, I tried to engage him in talking to the baby by laying his head on my belly. He acted like he felt silly but it opened up a conversation. He expressed concerns about being a father and knowing what to do. He didn't have a father growing up. His stepfather made it clear he was there for his mother but had no intention of being a father to either Jack or his sister. So Jack had no positive frame of reference for being a father. It was overwhelming to him at times, but I thought it would all work out once the baby came into the world.

Josh was born quickly, which was in line with his personality even today; he wastes no time once he makes a decision. I was in labor a mere two hours, barely enough time to get to the hospital and deliver, much less time to use my honed Lamaze breathing skills. He was two weeks early. Jack wanted to be in the room to count fingers and toes, but he hid behind a camera the entire time. He couldn't be present in the moment. I desperately needed for him to hold my hand, but he couldn't get that close. I begged him to put down the camera and join me at the bedside, but his fear prevented him from stepping into that circle of family. He stood back, filming the birth rather than experiencing the birth; it was a memory he found missing later in life when he needed it so much.

As our financial responsibilities increased, Jack acted more and more intense about little things—things I gave minimal attention until he exploded. Despite my confidence we were stable, he always felt like he was poor, like we would be on the streets any moment. He never carried cash and refused to use a debit card. Even then, checks were already almost obsolete, but he wrote checks for everything so he could keep a close accounting of the finances. It took an act of Congress for him to agree to buy something nice or go out to dinner. The true messiness of life and children unsettled him.

Inconsistent with his norm, when Josh was five months old, two years after we were married, Jack surprised me with a long-awaited honeymoon to Cozumel, Mexico. Sneakily, he arranged the trip with my work, and sprung it on me the day before we left. I was terrified at first! I couldn't imagine leaving our five-month-old baby and six-year-old and traveling out of the country for ten days.

As I pushed back, he said, "I need for you to trust me."

My trust had been challenged off and on since we married, not because he cheated, not because he was dishonest, but because I felt he never chose us. I didn't feel he had our back, so to speak. The very issue that bothered him about his own family played out in ours.

Jack arranged for David to stay with his grandmother and for one of my best friends, Joanne, to take care of Josh. Joanne and I had been pregnant at the same time. She had a baby girl who was four and a half months old, born only two weeks after Josh. We had thrived on the pregnancy news from each other all along the way. This was a gesture of pure love and friendship. Taking care of one five-month-old was enough, but two? Though I was extremely anxious about leaving Josh, I finally agreed.

We stayed in a house called Tortuga (or "Turtle" in English). It was a beautiful home with a diving board into the ocean. I remember the first dive we made there. Jack, among many other accomplishments, was a scuba diving master. He loved diving and had made the trip to Cozumel before we met many times. It was his way to escape the world. Under the water was one place he actually felt in total control. Because he was so detail oriented and I wasn't, I didn't quite share that sentiment.

Earlier in our marriage, I took a six-week diving course in the local swimming pool and became certified as a way to connect with him. This vacation was our first major diving trip and I was nervous. Not only was this uncharted territory, but I was also with a man I sometimes didn't trust.

While we were there, he was a different person in the water. It was as if he were my centurion, guardian, and teacher. He was patient and kind. He kept me above dangerous depths of water. Yet, he could also drop back and allow me to explore my new world, gently pulling up on my belt loops if I sank too deep or was unaware of impending danger.

We were carefree and reconnected on that trip in a way that sustained me for quite some time. He reemerged from that trip as the man I thought I married. The island seemed to ground him. He was far enough from the responsibilities of the mainland we could enjoy the moment.

It was a bizarre juxtaposition to everyday life as he became a carefree, confident, connected human being. He tolerated my need to call home often but seemed to want the freedom from family burdens. It pleased me to get the attention I so desired, but it concerned me he was so disconnected from our children.

I fell in love again on that trip. Needless to say, I had to hold on to those memories some days just to keep me sane. Despite leaving the children, I'm so glad we went.

* * *

When David was six, Jack coached little league soccer. When Josh was 13, Jack agreed to co-coach a flag football team to fulfill his duties as a father, and he was great at it. If he had a goal and he could conceive the plan, he executed that plan seamlessly.

However, Jack wasn't as up for the challenges of day-to-day living with the boys. If he felt rejected in any way, particularly when there were expressions of rebellion by the boys, he would remove himself for days, staying at work, or just disconnect from their emotional needs.

As is common with children when they feel safe, the boys would push back ("No!" or "I don't like you!") as a way of expressing discontent. Assuming their parents unconditionally loved them, they'd try out their rebellion in small ways, seeking more and more independence.

While it's healthy developmentally for children, it can be hurtful to us as parents because it brings up feelings of inadequacy. I often had to explain to Jack this was not rejection of him as a father but their outward need to claim independence in one way or another.

He couldn't grasp that idea. Rejection had been so painful for him in his life that neglect was actually more comprehensible, though frightening. So he sank deeply into work. He felt comfortable there because he could control his performance. He knew how to work. He knew how to please people in a work environment. He didn't know how to be a father.

Jack became remarkably more opinionated as time wore on and could put anyone on edge rather quickly with his acerbic nature. I gave way to his decisions most of the time because drama ensued if I disagreed. I learned quickly to choose my battles. He was bright and witty and when threatened could cut someone off at the knees with his words. He was on the offensive in most conversations. He behaved as if no one ever believed him, or believed in him. The rescuer in me only fought battles I thought were necessary and critical to the boys' or my welfare. Somewhere along the way, I realized I had given up a large part of my identity in the marriage while trying to play peacemaker.

The only aspect of our lives I insisted be kept separate was finances. He complained sometimes I never trusted him explicitly in the area of money. Ironically, throughout his career, he became a business expert and turned around large companies from failing to thriving, yet it was still an area of my life where I needed independence. I always wanted to work. I needed to work for my own well-being and I needed to be financially self-sufficient. He was very controlling in this area but I needed that freedom.

"Never rely on a man. Make your own money." My mother's words echoed in my head; I think she began telling me that the day I was born. Now I understand this philosophy was a reflection of her feelings of vulnerability, not her unhappiness. She worked some but very little, always unemployed because of the number of moves we made in the military. Logistically, I think she understood, but she also felt out of control as a military wife and mom, even though she was the controller of all household details.

I agreed to joint accounts in the first year of our marriage but one argument the first Easter about whether an Easter basket was "financially necessary" ended the enmeshing of monies. We split the bills from then onward so he couldn't question what I spent on the children. That's when, I believe, the separation of our lives began. Someone peering in from the outside could make the case we were never truly together as a family. There were only a few days I could have argued. It seemed his rationale was he couldn't step into the family if he couldn't control all aspects of our lives.

I once asked him if he missed the love and support of his family when he was at work for days at a time.

He said, "No. One doesn't miss what one doesn't know. If you don't know what you're missing, then how can you miss it?"

This construct was so foreign to me but gave me a picture of how he saw the world. He had adapted to his environment in a way that enabled him to function, but it slowly began to plague him. As he came to see the world from my perspective and through the lens of my experiences, he secretly wanted into step into the circle of family, but he just couldn't.

Consequently, he pulled further and further away in fear and into the financial success he was conditioned to value.

"In my family, you aren't a success unless you have respectable levels of education and financial status," he would say repeatedly through the years. "I don't know how to live in a family unit. It's not comfortable to me."

He wanted so much more but didn't have the resources to get it. He detached from the family because of fear; fear of failure, fear of making mistakes, fear of not being good enough, fear of not being loved.

There were other days I questioned if he could ever be part of a family because of his past. He was estranged from us most of the time. Neglect was all he knew, and in his mind, it was the lesser of two evils. However, I believe he longed for quite the opposite. I grieved often because all I wanted was to have a healthy, happy family. I couldn't be both mother and father to my kids. Had I made another ill-fated decision for my boys and me? I questioned it almost every day of my life with him.

The first several years of our marriage, our relationship was frequently strained. A flower in the desert eventually gives way to the elements. The erosion over time was painful, yet I stayed. We were both very busy with our careers and I was busy with the kids. We lived in a very nice area of town, we had a lovely house, and the kids went to the best schools. The demand to perform intensified. We hired a nanny to help me with the kids. I finished my master's degree and worked in the corporate health environment, but while accomplished, I was also lonely. Jack was gone most of the time. I felt overwhelmed and frenetic most days.

Finally, when I expressed my discontent with life, my level of stress, and the fact the kids never saw us, just like that, overnight, he put the house on the market and it was sold. We let go of the nanny and he had a plan to move us to a small town outside the city. I bought into the plan easily because I was exhausted.

To my ongoing shame, the nanny kept me informed of Josh and David's milestones in life and I was devastated I missed them. I really needed a break. I needed to be with my kids. I needed to spend time with them like I had before. I needed a husband who supported me emotionally.

"Maybe this is the answer," I thought.

We moved to a beautiful, small community outside the city. It had the charm of a fairy-tale book and the hospitality one would expect from a quaint town in Texas. I thought we were turning over a new leaf as a family, but what resulted was more of the same.

Less than a month after we moved, Jack announced he had bought into a business venture with two other guys he'd worked with previously. Unbeknownst to me, he had taken out a sizable loan to start a nonemergency transport business. Furious, I was helpless. I had no job and was now solely dependent on his income. I felt betrayed. I felt held hostage. The words of my mother haunted me at each turn.

What had I done? I knew no one there; the kids started school and I tried to fit in. It was a beautiful gated community on a golf course, but it was a retirement community and so many people had very different lifestyles. Instead of the guard at the gate protecting us from the outside, I felt trapped like a fish in a bowl. I resented Jack swung in now and then to throw us some fish food.

I met a few friends, most of whom worked, so I immersed myself in home projects and improvements. I would smother the boys when they came home from school, with questions and cookies ready! It was pathetic.

Miserable and unfulfilled, I decided to enroll in a PhD program to fill the void with school. The closest program was seventy-eight miles away. I got my master's degree at the same school and, while I knew it wasn't a good idea to leave, I moved on campus with Josh (who was five at the time), to work on my PhD. Jack supported my decision with a level of enthusiasm almost insulting to our relationship. He saw this as a solution to my ongoing discontent so he could focus on his business.

I registered Josh in kindergarten, and we lived in a seven-hundred-square-foot efficiency in bunk beds. David decided to try living with his biological father, so this seemed like a good time to keep my mind busy—busy thinking about education and achievement—and avoiding the pain of what was happening in my life.

My father and stepmother moved into our house and Jack lived out of his office. I had become him in some ways. I lived in a bubble on campus, focused on what I could control and ignored what I couldn't. It's amazing how quickly I sank into that behavior to protect myself from harm.

Jack maintained the house (I hesitate to call it home). He checked on my parents but lived out of his new company's office and nurtured the small, fledgling business twenty-four hours a day, seven days a week. We saw very little of one another. When we did see him, Jack showed more and more signs of manic behavior. The increase over time was subtle but, when this business became his life, he hardly slept or ate. I thought at the time anyone losing that much sleep would behave as erratically, so it was hard to know what was really going on. Maybe it was just a vicious cycle: work, no sleep, mania, no sleep, work, no sleep... and on and on.

Long days teaching at the university as a graduate teaching assistant, followed by long evenings as a single parent, followed by long nights studying three to five hours after Josh went to bed, proved exhausting. Exercise took a far backseat. As a matter of fact, I barely took a shower some days. There were days when I thought I'd give up. There were days when I wondered how long I could bear to be without David. While it was hard, thinking of David and Josh's futures drove me to hang in there. One day, I finally had a two-hour break in my schedule when I could make time to exercise. I needed it for stress reduction.

While clipping away on the treadmill, I caught up on the news. I witnessed the breach of the first World Trade Center tower and watched it burn. No one knew what was going on. The media was in a frenzy and the campus gym was silent. They switched all the televisions to the news. Each of us held our breath. Shock hung heavy in the room. Whispers overlapped like the gasps of an old steam engine just setting off from the depot. In the next few moments, the second plane crashed and the towers began to fall amid chaos and destruction. 9/11 is a day everyone will remember forever.

Life changed for families in the United States that day. There was so, so much senseless human loss. The aftermath also affected small businesses in America. The economy took a hard hit and many small businesses went under, as ours did, within two years after 9/11. This abruptly put my life into perspective.

Jack worked so hard at that business, but it failed. It wasn't due to neglect. After the terrorist attacks on the World Trade Center, insurance companies retracted significantly. Many decided his type of small business was too risky for them to insure. Losing the business was a devastating blow after all of his hard work. It crushed him, but after desperate attempts to save it, he eventually had to sell the business to his much larger competitor. He considered it a failure, and I don't think he ever recovered his confidence.

I worried he would take his life then. He threatened, but I just couldn't believe him. I dismissed the threats as a response to shock and worry. He'd put all of his heart and soul into this company he thought would make him millions. He thought his success would bring him the respect of his family, and then he would be loved and valued. We couldn't convince him he already was. He kept running from the demons of his childhood, when he was never good enough.

I studied long hours to earn a PhD in Public Health. David returned home, satisfied he'd found out what he needed to know about living with his father. The university I graduated from offered me a position and there was no doubt I should take it. Moving away from the area was not an option now. There was too much instability in the family, and David in particular needed stability. I couldn't bear to move him a long distance when he had just returned home. I took the position. We sold the house and moved the family to the university town permanently.

Desperately seeking employment, Jack went back to what he knew best: long hard hours in business, getting paid well, but working for someone else. It was as if he had to prove to himself even more now he was smarter and worked harder than everyone else. And he did.

Granted, Jack found another job, but I wondered whether we could ever truly start over. He'd suffered so much damage and loss it seemed he might never bounce back emotionally. Jack suffered with depression from losing the business, his success, the results of his hard work, and his autonomy. Again, he buried himself in work, refusing my help or the help of anyone else. He refused suggestions that he try counseling, therapy, medication, or just basic communication. He became very dark and difficult. Paranoia and anxiety began to creep out at night and dig in their claws into his being. He became more and more emotionally unavailable.

Contrary to my nature, I became resentful Jack would waltz in and out of our daily lives without a plan or intention. I desperately reached out to him in letters and emails as I became increasingly lonely and angry he was not seeking help.

David returned home a preteen after two years with his dad. There were distinct but expected challenges given his racing hormones, but he seemed happy. He found his group at school and seemed to hit his stride. Josh had a core group of friends he'd come to know well through school and sports. Both boys grew and thrived like they should. They seemed unfazed by Jack's absence. They also had their social lives separate from me.

I realized I was lonelier than I'd ever been in my life. I didn't really know who I was. I felt unneeded. My identity slipped away and yet I could feel the edge of the future with my outstretched fingertips.

4

THE RISE AND FALL OF THE VULNERABLE HUMANOID

JACK WAS AWAY SO MUCH of our marriage working, building and implementing new ideas, and gaining financial stability. When he was home, I felt mostly alone. I longed for him to step into the family circle, to go places and do things with us, to go on a vacation, or just be in the moment. To him, "being close" meant "observing from a distance." I would gently touch him on the shoulder some days and his entire body would physically jump as if his nerves had been caught unaware.

I never worried about unfaithfulness when he was away. His drive for success superseded any physical needs he had. In the twenty-plus years we were together, not once did he make a routine visit to a doctor or to a dentist. He always seemed healthy and had no physical problems at all. But he didn't get checkups or take supplements or medications.

Once in our years together he cut himself so deeply with a chain saw he agreed to go to the emergency room. Once sewn up, he was right back to overdrive, taking no pain medication for his injury. There were days when I asked him if he had been born an alien, or maybe he had robotic parts. It was obvious he had closed off his emotions and his physical needs. He worked like a machine and was very good at anything he set his mind to. He had occasional interpersonal disagreements with his superiors, but Jack's productivity at each company he worked for consistently trumped that of all other employees. The owners of his companies relished his achievements and soon he became well known in the industry for turning around failing businesses.

Unfortunately, over time he could not moderate his personal investment in corporate life. This was a part of his "all or nothing" mentality. Life was very black or white with no shades of gray. He either elevated people on a pedestal or they were his archrivals. There was seldom anything in between. The long hours of work drew him away from significant moments that would have built memories. He neglected important relationships and failed to build commitment and trust with people. Eventually, he said that he didn't feel worthy of self-care. This explained a lot about the course of our future.

Memories are the richness of the soul. It's in memories we learn what is good in our lives and what needs work. It's in memories we feel connected. Jack intentionally didn't build memories or relationships. Past experiences of failed connections brought him so much pain, disappointment, uncertainty, and fear he felt safer disconnected from people in his environment. This would harm him in the end.

Jack and I drifted apart little by little, becoming more like roommates than lovers. He said he didn't know how to be a part of our family emotionally, only financially. He knew how to make money. He didn't know how to be in a trusting, loving relationship, so he stayed away most of the time, occupying himself with fulfilling his financial obligations.

Now, in retrospect, I realize it was much too much to ask of this man to step into the circle of our family. Throughout our marriage I continued to invite him to all we did, to love him from a distance, but I went on many vacations alone with the boys. I became a "single" parent to the boys for most of their lives. To his credit, Jack would attempt to be a coach or a parent sponsor now and again—he could be an engaged partner when he was feeling successful at work—but he just wasn't there to make the memories. Memories take time, and time is not what he had for us. He spent his life running from his memories.

He didn't begin to change until his later years, when he felt more vulnerable. The fact decades had passed was remarkably meaningful and impactful for him. At forty, he began to have symptoms of frailties I had never observed in him. He seemed more fragile and more concerned about what others thought than I had ever realized.

Now I believe these fears were internalized as an extension of his childhood. He epitomized the façade of overconfidence and risky behaviors neglected children sometimes take on. But for some reason, he began verbally expressing them in a way that seemed almost paranoid. It didn't help he lost his business around this time. He found he had few resources to pull from his bag of tricks when the nonemergent transport business failed.

Until that point, he'd acted impervious to public opinion and lived his life in a devil-may-care fashion. People either liked him or were completely put off by him. Jack was clearly a presence to be managed. He could be loud and somewhat obnoxious. But there were many days the pendulum swung to the other extreme. He could be introverted, quiet, and triggered by mundane life events into panic and desperation quite easily.

After his uncertainties began to control him, we rarely went out with friends. When we did, he was the star of the show or he was the wallflower. There was nothing in between. He was racing or sleeping, boisterous or depressed, black or white, up or down. There were no shades of gray to this man.

I finally insisted we seek psychological help. In previous years, I attempted to solicit his participation in marriage counseling. To my disappointment, each counselor I engaged was reduced to rubble by the end of the session. Jack would completely (and actually quite impressively) frustrate and disarm them.

Jack explained he had no respect for psychologists and psychiatrists. He had very bad memories of being forced into counseling as a child by his exasperated mother and claimed he could outwit them even then. He didn't accept the suggestion they were there to help him, not hurt him. His childhood memory insisted counseling was just another means of reinforcing how bad he was.

"They were never interested in what I had to say," he scoffed. "My mother was paying for the sessions, so therefore, they were interested in making her happy, and I knew that at five years old."

As the days wore on, I felt like Jack was becoming more erratic. He would work long, hard hours as he was accustomed to, but he would also come home and sleep for the entire weekend. At the time, I attributed it to exhaustion; however, given his patterns through the years, I realize now it was probably depression. Holidays were always hard on him emotionally; he seemed to become considerably more antagonistic. He would announce prior to a holiday we would not buy presents for each other. While we were always secure financially, his growing sense of paranoia manifested in feelings of failure in family, business, and life.

We would have random conversations about purpose and the meaning of life, mostly without my contributions. He knew clearly what I believed. He would deliver monologues about what was factual and what was fairy tale as if he were trying to convince himself what he said was the truth. Each day seemed to be exponentially more stressful for him. I suggested he go back to school, seek out something new, or join me in church. Nothing seemed to satiate his restlessness.

It was then it dawned on me that he had no friends or hobbies. He had let everything he enjoyed be buried in the wake of his career. I encouraged him to make new friends, fly planes, or scuba dive as he had done before we were married. I filled my life with friends, hobbies, academia, and volunteerism, and I invited him to join. He would have none of it.

There was a chasm deep and wide between us for the thirteen years we'd been married. I felt like I had spent my life trying to build a bridge to his side, all the while fighting the fires he set to burn it down. It was exhausting and my energy was wearing thin. My health, both physical and mental, was in jeopardy. I decided it was time to leave.

I waited for David to graduate from high school and go to college before taking a permanent position. Until then, I just watched for jobs that could take me away.

I moved, on my own, several states away to Tennessee and felt completely liberated, though I don't know if it was truly liberation or just a false sense of freedom from worry. Exhaustion had consumed me.

Initially, I moved into a small apartment near the university. Jack had become increasingly demanding but more than that, his insecurities had begun to creep in as I found an advanced career and life of my own. He knew I was mentally checking out of the marriage. We agreed it might be wise not to take Josh out of school until I was sure I liked the area and would want to stay.

I thought the relationship was over and began to lead my life accordingly. I told Jack that I could not live the way I had been living for the last thirteen years and still have my health. My mother died very young and I'd had a number of breast scares myself through the years. I wasn't willing to risk the chance genetics, exacerbated by stress, would overtake my otherwise healthy body.

Separated, I thrived. I had time to breathe. I had time to think. As the fog lifted, it became clearer and clearer I had been living in an abusive, dysfunctional, and codependent relationship. Owning my contribution to it, I sought out counseling. I learned Reiki and self-care. My entire world, physically, intellectually, and spiritually, opened up like a time-lapse-photographed sunflower.

Josh followed me after a few months and we moved to a townhome. On the surface, Jack didn't seem upset. Knowing him as well as anyone, I suspected he felt overwhelmed to be caring for Josh alone. Once Josh moved to a place of "safety" with me, Jack probably felt relieved. He never trusted his judgement as a father.

The living spaces were much smaller than I was accustomed to but it was glorious. The position I held stimulated me. I put to use the time and energy leached away by my effort to maintain my relationship with Jack. Josh met friends his age, and he and I and went out to dinner with their families. We worked hard, but we also had laughter in the house again.

Before I knew it, two years passed. I found myself again. I made decisions without the battles and drama. We saw Jack some, but not often. He developed a fear of flying and, because the drive to see us was long, his visits were few and far between.

The increasing uncertainty in his life led to anxious conversations on the phone. In our second year of separation, he finally conceded our life together had been hard and he was willing to change. I knew how deeply ingrained his demons were, so I was skeptical and believed it was likely impossible for him to change, but there was an earnestness in his voice I had never heard. He knew he was losing the only person he felt had ever believed in him.

He was slow to apply to positions, but he finally accepted one. After nearly two and a half years of separation, he left his job and followed us to a new and culturally challenging city for him. In some ways, I thought, he was finding his way back to himself and trying to step into the circle.

5

HOPE RENEWED

FOR THE FIRST TIME IN ALL of my memory, he chose us. It was monumental for him, given his history. While he wasn't happy about the move and the new position was very challenging, he stepped in and he began to thrive. He had a clan, finally. He acted as if he had been on a respirator for years and was finally permitted to breathe on his own.

We moved into a house I loved; he agreed because its location was convenient to where he worked. David decided to transfer to the university where I taught, so Jack felt he had been given another chance with the boys. He participated in family events and seemed happy to be there. He engaged passionately with the boys and their interests—sometimes to their chagrin, because of the intensity with which Jack approached everything.

They needed time to get to know this person called Dad. They were occasionally awkward in their conversations with him, but they loved the opportunity of having a dad present. Though still somewhat emotionally distant, he began to move into the love we had offered him for so many years. He became "addicted," as he described it.

Not everything was coming up roses, but this flower began to flourish. He came home at a reasonable hour each day. He helped out around the house. Work went well and he seemed to be satisfied with the slower pace. He made unlikely friends along the way, friends who knew what a good guy he was. I was surprised to hear it. I knew he was a kind soul deep down, but we only saw hints of that now and again. To hear it from outsiders meant quite a lot to me.

We made friends with some couples. Not many, but a few. Very few people understood the intensity with which Jack lived his life and the intellect he wielded in conversations. However, these friends didn't seem to be bothered by the rambunctious, larger-than-life, extroverted personality that emerged from him in his new environment. I thought we finally had time to make some memories.

Jack began to actually live his life. He moved from a place of fear to what seemed to be a place of stability and comfort. The essence of his nature was unfurled beautifully and masterfully. He showed me and the kids affection. He hugged me in the morning and kissed me at night. Some evenings he sat in the kitchen and talked with me, helping with dinner. The transformation was remarkable; he was all-in. Or was he? There were still many days he seemed distant, restless, irritable, and worried about job-related issues, but overall he seemed to be "in."

I worried it was a ruse. How could I trust such a transformation in a short period of time?

* * *

Over the next few years, as part of a journey of personal exploration, I expanded my interest in and knowledge of the healing arts. I never took issue with integrating the natural and the supernatural. My ecumenical upbringing in the military and the beliefs passed down to me by my family allowed me the flexibility and curiosity to embrace the things that sometimes could not be explained.

I was rarely uncomfortable with other people's perspectives, and I could support other people's beliefs, even if they weren't necessarily my own. I taught full-time at a university and worked with people who had experienced war trauma. I worked with refugees and veterans. My research attempted to understand why some people adjust well in the aftermath and others do not.

Western-style medical treatments have limitations. Holistic healing practices, like hypnosis, meditation, and other energy modalities, drew my interest.

I have always been a deeply spiritual person and believed God was leading me down this path. I learned rapidly and earned certifications in a number of alternative healing practices, to be used alongside my academic training. I felt compelled to do more integrative practice in my work with war-related trauma. I asked Jack if he thought I could make a business work well enough to leave the tumultuous department at the university.

Jack was respectful. He said, "That's your thing, not mine. But go for it!" We put steps in place to make it work. I began seeing clients and over the course of only a year, my practice reached capacity. My life path seemed to be snapping into place. I was really happy running a business, seeing clients, consulting in academia, and having a relatively stable home life.

Interestingly, during this time and without persuasion, Jack developed a curiosity about spirituality. He began to read books he'd never imagined existed by such authors as Wayne Dyer and Eckhart Tolle. It was so humorous to watch his amazement there were books out there he didn't know about. He would say things like, "I can see what I've missed" and "I've missed so much, haven't I?"

We began to forge a relationship we'd never had before. There were glints of the past now and then, but the cadence of our relationship was much more balanced. It was incredible we had evolved to this place in our careers and our marriage in such a short period of time. I thought often about what could have been the catalyst for the change.

6

TRUSTING

AS QUICKLY AS HE BECAME committed and engaged, Jack became progressively more agitated and anxious. It was as if his light had been doused overnight and darkness swallowed him. Over the course of a few months, he reverted back to many of his old habits. For two years, he had seemed to be all-in; now I was perplexed he could so easily revert back to being a person we weren't sure we even liked.

Jack had become a high performer in his own job and I believed he was bored. He needed a new challenge. Jack never did well when he felt like he was trapped in a box. He needed something new, or at least to be able to progress in his current position.

Jack began dropping comments randomly about his regional supervisor. He didn't think this supervisor was happy with him. A driving force behind Jack's actions in business was his desire to avoid making important people in his work life disappointed in him at all cost (and many times to the detriment of his personal life). He would do anything within his power to keep those people happy—unless he couldn't. Then he would remove himself from the situation or quit. In this case, he couldn't leave the company. We depended exclusively on his benefits since I had moved into being a small business owner and consultant. He felt boxed in.

As was the case with other companies Jack worked for, I got the sense his boss wasn't happy unless there was a steady increase in sales. The catch-22 about Jack's work ethic was as hard as he worked his company always wanted more. When he began his job by running a marathon for the company, then they would expect a double marathon the next year. By year four, Jack had maximized the company's production for its size and the resources with which he had to work. He could not increase production unless there was a remarkable investment in a particular part of that company. The company wasn't willing to do that. To his disadvantage, Jack never developed a personal connection or relationship with his boss—that was hard for him to do. He felt his back was against the wall. He was also approaching his fiftieth birthday and these milestone birthdays were peculiarly hard on him.

It was obvious he felt vulnerable and searched for other answers in life. He would begin conversations by saying, "There has to be more to all of this. We are much more than robots, slogging away to make money for big business, aren't we?"

Recognizing he was searching for a higher meaning or purpose for being human, I would simply say, "Yes." I'd learned if I continued, he lost interest. If I simply answered with a yes or no, the conversation would continue.

Knowing my positions on God and spirituality, he began to ask interesting questions, like, "Do you think we've been together before in another lifetime?" or "Do you think we'll be together again in another lifetime?" I thought it was quite curious because over our time together, he'd had little use for religion or spirituality.

While we were dating, I told him my greatest concern about marrying him was he didn't know what he believed. Spirituality was very important to me. He bantered about physics and science. He claimed to be a Christian agnostic, a term with which I had no experience. He quoted Hawking, Feynman, Einstein, and Darwin. And yet, daily, he would now ask me these types of questions.

I gave him books I had read through the years and he read them, sometimes in a day. A prolific reader, he confessed he never knew some of the concepts in my books existed. He would seek out more to read and research spiritual topics in which he was interested. He sought out information on God and the afterlife, reading my books on hypnosis and patients' experiences with past lives under hypnosis.

Then we would have conversations about love and acceptance, views of different religions and their concepts. He began watching television ministers with an insatiable curiosity. Jack had always been "all or nothing" in most aspects of his life, so while I was pleased he had opened up to other possibilities, I wasn't surprised by his fervor. He continued on this rapid path of spiritual transformation.

As I reflect back on these days, I realize for a person who lived his life like a satellite, sending out signals out and hoping for a response, these spiritual concepts were probably difficult to integrate once he learned about them. There was a chasm of time and space between his understanding and his ability to apply these ideas.

All the while, he became more and more agitated. Sometimes he seemed paranoid about his work situation. He frequently conveyed what I thought were unfounded concerns he would lose his job soon.

"Be positive. You're only imagining all of this," I said, trying to encourage him. How could a company fire a regional manager who had turned the business from one that had suffered gross losses to one of the top performers in the nation? It was quite confusing to me and reinforced my thoughts he was being paranoid again.

One dark and gloomy evening, rain moved in and mist hung in the air. I was in the kitchen making dinner when he came home and announced he had been let go from his position. He began to cry. I was in shock. I had never seen this man cry, even when he fell out of a tree and almost severed his arm from his body with a chain saw.

The business, while not a sexy one, was one Jack was very proud of—one he had prevented from going down in flames like the *Hindenburg*. They let him go at age fifty, in a very cruel and unexpected way... and yet, with his stuffing lying on the floor, he reminded me it was just business as usual. Over the years, he had worked his way up through the ranks to manage regions with large numbers of employees. He was good at this. He had education, money, and business success, and life was good—until one day it all stopped. The dream he had built popped like a big red balloon at a birthday party. Something unimaginable happened that day. Something seemed to change him at the soul level.

I had seen glimpses of what he was capable of conjuring up in his head, but this was a side of him that was too paralyzed to move ahead. He was a man whose very integrity had been questioned, and he would be replaced by someone much younger and paid half the salary. So many days, he would recount events in his mind. He would roll them over like clay in a potter's hands —searching for answers about what went wrong.

Jack was never the same after that day. We embraced and we cried together. I assured him it would all be okay—because it always was. Tragically, from that day forward, he became fearful of everything. Fearful he would never work again, but mostly fearful I would leave him. I trusted everything would be okay, but what the unconditional love I claimed caused me to endure was staggering. I felt like a hypocrite some days.

To love unconditionally means to love like there are no conditions around that love, no strings attached. Jack needed unconditional love, as we all do, from someone—anyone. I questioned my ability to do that day in and day out. I taught this concept in workshops and private sessions for clients and yet, I struggled.

As he became more anxious and seemed to be spinning out of control, I asked myself, "Where is the line between unconditional love and subconsciously enabling behaviors?" I realized I just didn't know.

Deflated entirely by his firing, Jack and I began to strategize about how to keep us afloat. While my business was thriving, it couldn't possibly replace his salary. We also needed to secure health benefits until he found his next position. With a track record like he had in business, he was highly marketable. While still employed, several other companies tried to recruit him, so I believed this would be an easy rebound. Unfortunately, he didn't believe it.

Struggling to recover, Jack applied to many companies. He got many calls and many phone interviews but nothing worked out. He'd had the stuffing knocked out of him, but I felt he would be in full swing within weeks. He was amazing at rebounding. It was what he did for companies, and now I had no question that he could do it for himself.

By Thanksgiving, he was frustrated. He had become more distant and agitated. He read voraciously. He kept reminding me the holiday season was not a good time to be looking for a job. He slept a lot. I took on more clients than I had been taking and consulted for two universities. Financially, we were fine, but I could feel him slipping away.

By Christmas, he was obviously depressed. I tried to pull him out of the quicksand of sorrow he seemed to be voluntarily slipping into. I encouraged him to think about going back to school again. He loved knowledge, studying, and books. He'd always lamented he didn't get his PhD after his master's.

"Jack, help me help you. What should we do to prepare you to get back out there?" I begged.

"Nothing," he snapped back. "The market is just tough right now."

While I understood that to be true, I also knew there was no stopping this guy when he put his mind to something. We minimized our spending for Christmas and I secured a health insurance policy. There were no issues paying bills, but the level of anxiety he felt was palpable. There were several calls from potential employers; I'm not sure why nothing panned out. I began to think he was self-sabotaging. I asked him frequently about whether he was actually going to interviews. He rarely responded. He had sunk pretty low.

To lift his spirits and reposition him for optimism, I remarked, "The holidays are a tough time to get a job anyway. The first of the year will be a golden opportunity. Hang in there and it will all work out to your advantage." He rested and read, but nothing much else.

After the first of the year, an opportunity came forth and he made it through the first three interviews. I had never known him to be nervous, but he was remarkably shaken by each interview. They told him he had the position but they wanted to fly him to headquarters to meet the president of the company. He unraveled. The fear of flying he developed haunted him. He was terrified to get on a plane. Or maybe it was a fear of being away from home, or a fear of not being able to hold it together at the interview. I suspect it may have been a combination of them all.

In his younger days, he had bungee-jumped, scaled mountains, and flown planes. All of that stopped after we married. Early in our marriage, he spent 80 percent of his time on a plane for work purposes. Now the thought of flying paralyzed him. It was only symptomatic of things to come.

He called me after the flight when he arrived at the hotel. He said he made it. He didn't mention much about how he did on the plane, he just told me he was a wreck when he was picked up by the company at the airport. I imagined he didn't do well; that he ruminated on every little detail of his firing (as he had before he left), and then worked himself up into a frenzy by the time he landed.

He returned from the interview with a feeling he wouldn't be offered the job. He wasn't. I never knew why. He wouldn't talk about it. I got the sense he may not have interviewed well. Maybe he had a panic attack before he walked in. Or possibly they were just looking for someone else. I'll never know.

I knew I had to keep encouraging him to get back out there, but he would barely leave the house anymore. What had happened to this man who took the corporate world by storm and took no prisoners? What happened to the man who revived failing companies and made them thrive? Why could he not apply this business strategy to his own life?

7

THE DAY IN THE WOODS

THE GUN TREMBLED IN JACK'S HAND. I shouted his name again and his eyes locked on mine. We held eye contact for several thudding heartbeats.

He laid the gun in the grass beside him. He moved simultaneously like a child and an old man, clumsy and slow. He cowered, eyes to the ground, as if he were ashamed. He looked frail and desperate.

He eyed the gun on the ground like it represented his freedom slipping away. Disappointment clouded his face. He had been mere moments from eternal rest when my shouting shattered his peace in an instant.

He shuffled to me, limp, like a lifeless zombie. I shook as if I had a raging fever. I repeated—softly but loud enough for him to hear—what sounded like a singsong lullaby: "Come to me. Keep walking; keep walking... Come to me."

He emerged from the woods trembling, innocence washing over his face. We both shook, but our shivers came from very different reactions.

When he reached me, he surrendered to my care. I took other, lesser weapons from him. I guess he felt if he lost the will to use one, he would try another. My heart hurt; the pain deep and sadness overwhelming. The weight of the world pressed on us.

We stumbled into the house. I dragged a chair into the middle of the room, far from anything that could harm him. It engulfed him, a broken man, this man I lived with, whom I would love and nurture until death did us part.

As Jack sat in the chair, defeated and trembling, I called the local crisis center. I had the number at hand, left over from my arduous and desperate search for an open psychiatric practice.

For the past couple of months, as his depression escalated, I called every psychiatric/psychological resource I could find in the area. Most were closed to new patients.

After living in a city of 250,000 people for nearly five years, I'd discovered a disgusting shortage of professional psychologists and psychiatrists.

Jack urgently needed help. Watching him deteriorate so quickly was not only unnerving but also uncharted territory for me. Initially, no one would or could accept him as a patient. Instead, we were placed on waiting lists. Physicians whose practices weren't closed to new patients were booking appointments as far out as six weeks, sometimes more. Psychologists in the area had similar waiting lists. Incredibly, I secured an appointment three weeks away with a psychiatrist who, unfortunately, had poor reviews, but we had no choice.

As in many cities across the nation, a major psychiatric hospital serving our community closed three years prior. Many professionals left the area. The local shortage of practitioners became critical.

The crisis center answered after one ring. I explained what just happened and said it was critical he be assisted as soon as possible. They informed me there were no beds available in the city and told me to wait for twenty-four hours. They expected to have one available the next day.

I hung up, frustrated and angry I could not get this man the timely assistance he needed. Within the last hour, Jack successfully drained the last ounce of my steam (or so I thought). We were in crisis. Isn't that what a crisis center was commissioned to manage?

I walked Jack into the room where he had been sleeping for the last few months. He rarely slept with me during our marriage, but now it was nearly impossible. Since childhood, he needed to sleep with a light on and with background noise. Most nights he slept on the leather couch in the den with the dogs. He was most comfortable there.

He told me he rarely slept in a bed as a child. When asked why, he could never explain. I suppose this may have been one of the indicators of the deep insecurity and fear he masked through the years, but I accepted it. He always worked long and unusual hours. When he slept at home, he needed the alarm clock to sound with the intensity of a fire engine siren to wake him.

After being let go, he became so restless at night I couldn't sleep with him either. He retreated to another bedroom in the house. I lay next to him with my hand on his back and he fell asleep. Overcome with grief, I tried to return to my work.

That evening he had one panic attack after another. He began chattering nonsensically, eyes wild and darting. I called the crisis center again and they advised I take him to the emergency room. I knew an emergency room visit might mean he would be taken involuntarily to a psychiatric hospital.

Though I was in full agreement with their recommendation, it would be nearly impossible to convince someone who was six foot two, two hundred pounds, and experiencing paranoia and panic, to get in the car and go to the emergency room. I felt he just needed some short-term assistance and if it came in the form of a hospital stay, I was all for it. But Jack was convinced if he ever went into the hospital, he would never get out. There was no persuading him.

That night, I insisted he sleep in the bed with me so I could keep a hand on him. I fought hard to stay awake, to hold on to him and to keep him alive. Generally, I would awaken to the sound of his breath. Exhausted, I eventually fell into a state of sleep deeper than any I ever remembered experiencing.

* * *

The next morning, I awoke with alarm. Jack wasn't in bed.

I jumped up and scrambled into the den, where I found him rapidly pacing. He circled the room like a marble in a bowl. Repeating relentlessly his brain was not right, he pleaded with me to help him leave his body behind. He emphasized I just couldn't understand the pain he felt all over his body.

I succumbed to a calmness induced by my exhaustion and adrenal depletion. I whispered he needed medication and if he went with me to the emergency room, we would get him something for anxiety. I couldn't just focus on the fact we needed him as a family. That always caused his condition to escalate within seconds, drudging up feelings of inadequacy and his sense he was failing at his responsibilities. I reassured him we all needed him to stay with us and that we would be very sad if he left.

I hadn't seen his anxiety heightened to this level before. His emotional state cycled between fear, anger, frustration, exasperation, and sheer panic. I walked with him as he paced, but he wouldn't let me touch him. He flinched and twitched as if intermittent electric shocks peppered his back and shoulders. He told me his skin was crawling and it just wouldn't stop.

I had never known panic like this. I had never felt it; I had never seen it. His face flushed and his eyes bulged, as if his fear literally held him by the throat. After several loops around the room, he finally agreed to allow me to take him to the emergency room, but only to get a prescription for antianxiety medication.

This was a monumental decision on his part. Again, he had never taken even an aspirin to my knowledge. He'd mostly managed the chemical imbalances he experienced through the years with diet, intensive exercise, and immersion in his work. He would never consent to taking medication, sometimes at the expense of those around him. The very fact he had agreed to do so now told me he knew this was serious and unmanageable for him. For me, his concession was a relief.

Quietly, I gathered a few things, anticipating that he might stay in the hospital a day or two. Jack believed we would go in to get a prescription and come home. Truly not knowing what would be the end result of the day, I let him believe we would be returning home in a matter of hours.

We arrived at the emergency room and with one look at the both of us, nurses at the front desk hopped into action. Within minutes, they escorted us to a room. After they established my level of concern for his well-being, they took us down the hall and locked in a room that appeared to have been recently washed with bright white paint.

It contained a bed with white sheets and little else. They took his shoes, belt, and other personal items they perceived to be a threat. Jack fell onto the bed as if he were home. The surreal nature of his calm demeanor toyed with my patience. Incredibly, I saw him transform in front of my very eyes. As he lay there in a state of steadiness, my adrenaline-drenched emotions raged. But I had to keep it together, one more time.

After hours of waiting, we met with the doctor. He was cordial and young, and obviously in a hurry. He explained Jack would have a psychiatric consult by a nurse and his fate would be determined from there.

Another hour passed and a chaplain arrived to talk with Jack about his state of mind. While very nice, the chaplain seemed to be there more for me than for Jack. I appreciated his kindness. His gentle voice was calming and effective. As he continued, the door opened and a television monitor rolled into the room.

The chaplain explained a nurse, in some remote location, would carry out the psychiatric evaluation, appearing on the screen to ask her patient critical questions. The chaplain exited and left us alone with her image on the monitor.

I'd seen this process performed in small rural hospitals when I worked in the public health field. In an attempt to cut costs across the nation, hospitals introduced "telemedicine" as an alternative to hiring a full-time employee to interact with patients. This method does give people in remote and underserved areas areas better access, but it's remarkably impersonal. At the time, I couldn't comprehend how this was Jack's best access. We lived in a city of 250,000 people. It was hardly rural.

I understand tele-interviews have become standard for many hospitals due to a shortage of personnel working in psychiatry, but the irony is profound. When people in this condition need a human to validate their existence so desperately, the impersonal nature of the interaction is a cruel blow.

I had very few resources left in my repertoire. The lack of sensitivity inherent in this method of psychiatric interview left me impatient and irritable.

As the nurse began her evaluation, we could only see the side of her face because of where she'd positioned her monitor in relation to the camera. She appeared never to be looking at Jack.

I stopped her for a moment and asked, "Is this the way you intend to evaluate a person who is in extreme mental distress?"

She nodded. This was the way the hospital did all psychiatric evaluations.

"Can you please at least look at him?" I struggled to contain my anger.

She didn't. She continued her evaluation looking into her monitor, away from the camera.

A patient in crisis needs to feel he is important enough to be seen. I felt Jack's sadness growing. What he had thought would be a solution to his problem was turning out to be even more isolating. Desperate for any form of a solution, I let her continue.

The nurse finished up her inquiry. Her rubric indicated a need for admission to a psychiatric hospital for observation, so she began the process of involuntarily admitting him for suicide watch.

His body relaxed into what appeared to be resolve, relief, or maybe just defeat. He rested deeply without medication, his face serene and childlike. As he dozed off, I stared down at him with a heavy heart. I felt I had betrayed him. As tears welled in my eyes, he could feel my pain.

He slowly opened his eyes and whispered, "You know, I will never come out, but it's not your fault. I know you love me."

A dagger to the heart could not have been more painful. Yes, I deceived him for what I thought was his own good. All I could do was muster my ability to dissociate from the pain and trust I was doing the right thing for him.

An unfamiliar nurse waddled in and asked me to leave the room. Her pen scratched a staccato rhythm on the paperwork she flipped through. Jack gave me a look of approval and I reluctantly stepped out.

My mind spun as I leaned against the hard, unforgiving wall outside of his door. The alarms and the beeping of medical electronics in the emergency unit reverberated obnoxiously in my head. I had so many things to consider.

How had we gotten here? How could life as we knew it change seemingly just overnight? Or had it happened that fast? In actuality, our condition had gradually morphed a bit each day, as if we were frogs in a pot of water on the stove, the heat rising unnoticeably until it became lethal.

They prepared to move him. A police officer arrived and stepped confidently past me and into the room. He closed the door, but I leaned against it to listen. I could only hear the mumblings of abrupt directions being given to Jack. I had to catch myself when the door opened. The police officer led Jack out, handcuffed.

Slumped and humiliated, he lumbered into the hallway, shuffling in tennis shoes with the laces removed. This broken man was not the business powerhouse I remembered from the early years of our marriage. He locked his begging and defeated eyes on me, and they pierced me like spears.

Furious and feeling tears beginning to well, I burst out, "He's not a criminal! He's just ill. He's not violent! Take him out of those cuffs... Please!" A river of tears I couldn't stop streamed down my face.

I sobbed, my chest caving in with each breath. I could barely see through the fog of tears clouding my eyes. I couldn't fathom why they would handcuff an otherwise brilliant and nonviolent man.

Jack barely managed to say, "It's okay. It will be all right."

As they filed past me, the police officer cut in. "He *is* a threat, ma'am. He's a threat to himself. I'm sorry, but you can't go with him."

The officer turned quickly, one hand leading Jack by the arm, and they disappeared down a set of stairs.

I turned; looking for any kind or familiar face to tell me what was happening. The hallway began to spin. Tunnel vision encroached on my ability to recognize anyone who had been in the room. I shook my head to regain awareness. I whispered under my breath, "*Please*, God, just not like this."

Finally, a nurse arrived with information about his admission to a local hospital. I signed paperwork they gave me a set of instructions for family members. The tears that kept flowing were an annoyance. I needed to pay attention to when I could see him next, the articles of clothing and personal items he could have, and other important information. I didn't have time to cry.

Thankfully, she handed me a page of instructions and a list of rules. I couldn't comprehend what else she said. Her voice had a hollow sound, like a voice calling your name when you're deep asleep.

Stunned, I staggered to my car, steadying myself against the hallway wall along the way, alone. As I sat in the car, I read the rules. I could bring shoes or slippers with no laces, pants with no strings, ties, or belts. I could bring up to two books or magazines. All other personal supplies would be provided. I could only see him for thirty minutes twice during the week. What had our life been reduced to?

I hoped this was just the beginning of help and healing. I clung to that idea.

8

DYSTOPIA

THE HOSPITAL STRICTLY LIMITED visitation and Jack could make only one call each day. He chose not to call the first two days. I longed for him to call, but I understood his silence.

Family members called from out of state, offering a tidal wave of recommendations and assistance. I really didn't know what we needed. Jack needed a new brain, new chemistry, a new body maybe; nothing else seemed relevant or important.

The hospital looked institutional. True, it was the only hospital with a bed available, but more than that, it was the only one the system thought we could afford.

We had been blessed to have medical insurance the entire twenty years we were married. We hardly used it except for well checkups—even for the children. However, because Jack was unemployed and I was an independent contractor, we now paid high premiums for individual insurance and had no coverage for behavioral health. Therefore, we were considered uninsured.

The staff was cordial but very busy and unresponsive. I arrived shortly after I composed myself, armed with basic items for his survival in the hospital.

The facilities seemed clean, but it felt like the clocks had stopped ticking sometime during the 1960s or '70s. Mass-printed pictures donned taupe walls. I remembered many from doctor's offices I'd seen as a child. A familiar print of a guardian angel walking children across a bridge hung in the waiting room. The same print used to hang in a bedroom at my grandmother's house; it comforted me then. As an adult, in this setting, I felt nauseated.

I turned over his personal items for inspection. They only allowed him two books at a time. They didn't know Jack would finish a book a day, and my next visitation was not for four days. I hoped he could have an extra book until I could bring others. They didn't allow it. They returned the third book to me. Once they cleared everything else, they took his items away and I left. I felt eerily hopeful. I needed to have hope; it was all I had.

My mind frequently drifted to my children. Thankfully, our youngest son was at Boy Scout camp over a long weekend. I was so grateful he hadn't experienced this event. David had already graduated from college and moved to Nebraska for his first job. Both of them knew Jack struggled with depression and were aware of pieces leading up to this moment, but neither of them knew about the weekend's events yet.

Jack spent seven days under suicide watch. Each day I called and left messages with his case manager. I called several times a day, but no one was available to speak with me. I received a call from his consulting psychiatrist on his second day at the hospital, and he asked me a number of questions about Jack's family history of mental illness and relevant questions about his behavior. This conversation was brief and specific to the doctor's inquiry. Any questions I began to ask were interrupted with a pat response. He said a case manager would call and update me on his progress.

Social workers were responsible for calling family members with updates, but their workload was overwhelming. To get any information at all, I called the evening shift and spoke with a receptionist who, when given a password, would read his treatment notes for the day from a computer. I learned he'd seen a psychiatrist that week for two visits of about five minutes each, and he'd been diagnosed with bipolar disorder.

By the third day, Jack called and begged me to pick him up. He couldn't bear the solitude, the boredom, or the screams through the night. He said he paced the halls all day with one of the books I had left with the front desk. The mental conditions of the two to three people housed in his room varied but were mostly severe.

He said people were obviously "drugged up" and senselessly babbled and screamed all night. Most distressing was a nightmarish darkness about the place that overlaid the haunting screams and groans at night. He felt the stay was torturous. He claimed being away from his family was killing him. I found it ironic he made this claim. Choosing to take his life would remove him from his family permanently. The solitude, the boredom, and the disruptions in sleep were only conditions of his living.

Finally, on the fourth day of his stay, after what seemed to be a lifetime, a good friend, Steve, and I arrived at the hospital along with other people bringing staple items for distressed family members. At precisely four p.m., they gathered us in a hallway and gave specific and detailed instructions of what was and what was not permitted for the visit. "Institutional" again came to mind as we stood elbow to elbow in the dimly lit hallway; one attendant lead the group and one followed.

Somber, they herded us down a long corridor. The group flinched at each faint yell or scream coming from behind a closed door. They assured us our family members were not housed with other patients experiencing more distress, but the screams were unsettling for everyone. As we wound our way deeper into the hospital, I felt sicker each time we passed through a partitioned and locked section of the hallway.

Double doors opened to a large cafeteria-style visiting area. They asked us to find a seat at a table and informed us our loved ones would join us soon. Steve filled the pregnant minutes. His positive presence uplifted me in this otherwise abysmal situation. He encouraged me and gave me a sense of support I so desperately needed.

Jack entered the room. He seemed calm. I knew with Steve at the table, he would remain calm. Jack measured his behavior in front of other people, as he had with me during the majority of our lives together. Over the last two years, he had less control over his behavior around me, but still maintained a stance of confidence with friends and family.

Inextricably, I had always associated Jack's mind with strength and control. In our early years together, he seemed to control his thoughts and behaviors like no other person I knew. His relentless drive for perfection was hard on the family at times, but it's what I believed made him so successful in his career.

In the end, it was a coping mechanism a ruse—and one that made him so vulnerable. Through the years, I tried to instill in him my belief perfection is unattainable and a contradiction to living. To me, perfection meant there was no room for improvement, which is impossible.

After several minutes, Steve excused himself so Jack and I could speak privately. Almost immediately, Jack began to beg to leave. The characteristics of his illness manifested right in front of me. I remember thinking some of this might be an act he'd reserved for me, but why would someone go to this extent? How could Jack manage so well in front of a friend and then fall apart upon his departure? It was all so frustrating.

"What medications have they started for you?" I asked.

"None yet," he said, almost boastfully. "I told them I don't want any medications." While he'd initially been open to medications while in crisis, he'd cycled back to our daily struggles around medications.

"Jack, after what we've just experienced, you can't come home without something!" Coming from a person like me, who practiced alternative therapies and avoided medication until it was the last resort, this was significant.

The case manager joined the table within minutes. I asked why he had not been given medication.

She explained though he had been involuntarily admitted, he had a choice about taking medication.

I was stunned. I felt my throat closing up, and my voice became higher pitched. "*He* has a choice?" I began to tremble.

"Yes, he has a choice." Shaking her head, she repeated, "He has a choice."

Turning to Jack, I began to cry. I begged him to at least try something because I couldn't bear an experience like the one we'd had earlier in the week.

Reluctantly, he agreed. The case manager made notes and our time was up.

It seemed like those thirty minutes had moved at warp speed. I was thankful I could only visit once; I wasn't sure if I could even make it back home after the experience. I couldn't imagine what it would be like to be a patient there. I still can't.

* * *

They discharged Jack after seven days with three prescriptions and no follow-up appointment scheduled.

I called the prescribing psychiatrist's office and his staff told me if the physician saw Jack outside of the hospital, it would be considered a conflict of interest and breach of contract by the hospital. Yet, the hospital had no recommendations for his follow-up care.

We were back in the same position we had been in before he was admitted. His mental state and demeanor were unchanged and now were compounded by the intolerable side effects of some of his medications.

9

AFTER THE ADMISSION

THE DAYS LEADING UP TO Jack's admission to the hospital had been surreal. The hospital experience had been a nightmare. And now, Jack had been released from the hospital on a Friday, and I had a three-day interview scheduled to begin Sunday at a university three hours away.

I had to find a place of financial stability with health benefits. Recognizing our financial reserves couldn't hold up in the face of bills like the $9,000 one we received from the hospital, I had applied to a position at a university. But now, sleep deprived and emotionally a wreck, I panicked at the thought of leaving Jack at home, and even more so at the thought of taking him with me.

Jack had been a mostly responsible father when he was home, but he just wasn't himself now. I wouldn't leave Josh alone with him. But I couldn't think of anyone in town whom I wanted to tell or burden with this issue. David had just graduated from college and moved to another state for a job. I couldn't ask him to come home now.

I had to get to that interview. I called Jack's father and begged him to fly in from Dallas to help me. I had no other choice. Barry agreed to fly in and stay while I bolted to the interview.

"God help me," I thought. "I can't possibly pull this off."

I asked Barry to come in a day early so I could get some sleep, but I hadn't prepared a lecture or research presentation. I had three days of interviewing ahead of me and my brain barely functioned.

I arrived at the hotel on Saturday about three p.m. I promptly turned off the light, lay down, and slept for twenty hours.

The three-day interview process began Sunday night with dinner. Until then, I worked on my presentations. I recall very little about those days, other than remarkably kind faculty and staff. The experience feels surreal, like a dream.

When I returned home, Jack's spirits seemed to have lifted. He enjoyed his father's attention. Over the years, Jack's father had shared the remorse he felt about leaving Jack and his sister. Apologies can never mend the past, but they go a long way to heal the future.

Jack's father stayed a couple more days. I was still shaken by the distress of the previous week. Barry's presence gave me enough support to feel maybe these days were only temporary and we'd make it through. I was very thankful to have him there.

The following week, the university offered me the position I'd interviewed for. I accepted.

I cried after I hung up the phone. When you're struggling through darkness, small breaks become really big. I was overcome with gratitude. What a gift.

As with many positions in academia, although I signed my contract in February, my job wouldn't begin until August. This meant we had several months for Jack to heal. I planned to get a small apartment and commute there each week. Things seemed to be looking much better.

* * *

After his discharge from the hospital, Jack took strong medications for depression, anxiety, and bipolar disorder. To this day, I still question the diagnosis. It seemed at the time everyone I talked with had a diagnosis of bipolar disorder. It was very disconcerting. Although his family had a genetic history sprinkled heavily with depression and bipolar diagnoses, it seemed so unlikely to me someone would develop bipolar disorder at fifty years of age. I waffled between believing he had always been bipolar, resulting in his erratic behaviors through the years, or if he was just broken in spirit.

To add insult to injury, we still couldn't get an appointment *anywhere* for four weeks after discharge. We went on a waiting list for three physicians.

He remained at home in a very fragile state. Some days he didn't get up to eat. In my estimation, he was dying, a slow and cruel death.

He began having more and more persistent and excruciating pain all over his body. I was livid I couldn't get access to health care for him. I rolled over in my mind what to do. I wasn't willing to wait for the appointment.

I called mental health practices around large cities where we had family located. I thought we could get him into a practice more easily in a larger city. I was wrong. It was almost as difficult.

I found one physician willing to take Jack as early as Sunday (yes, Sunday) in the Dallas–Fort Worth area. This psychiatrist had a cash-only, no-insurance practice and charged $450 for an evaluation and $375 per hour.

Shell-shocked by the charges and knowing this might be a several-week proposition, I took a deep breath. We had to do this. We had no choice. I could not imagine Jack going four weeks without treatment.

"How do people who don't have the financial means get treated?" I thought.

Jack's parents gladly helped with the expenses incurred at the hospital, so I felt this was doable. We had access to retirement accounts, what was left of our savings accounts, and family members who could help. I felt blessed, but I was angry the "system" had us by the throat.

I booked Jack's flight to Dallas for the next day. Something inside me braced for the fact it might take a long time for him to recover.

Barry lived within 45 minutes of the psychiatrist's office. I called and asked him to pick Jack up at the airport and bring him to the appointment.

When I arrived at the airport with Jack, I grew increasingly concerned about his ability to fly. I worried about the ethics of putting him on the plane in the first place. Because he was now afraid of flying, I had visions of him melting down under pressure up in the air.

He assured me he had taken his medications, including the Xanax for anxiety. He seemed fairly relaxed and lucid. I went as far through the check-in and bag-check lines as I possibly could, reassuring him we were on the way to finding help.

My mind kept drifting back to my watch. In the midst of all of this, I was the lead person on a committee to distribute grant funds to a number of organizations. In denial, I suppose, I assumed I could push through the process. In some ways, it gave me a necessary distraction and a sense of normalcy I so desperately needed.

I sped from the airport back to the final allocation meeting. After making the thirty-mile trek, I received a call from Jack as I pulled into the parking lot of the nonprofit foundation.

"The flight was canceled due to weather in Atlanta," he said with an arrogant tone. Part of me felt he was mocking me—and my efforts to get him help. My head began to swirl. He told he hailed a cab and would arrive home within the hour.

My mind raced. "What should I do?" I panicked for a moment. Our sixteen-year-old son was home alone and I would not be home from this meeting for three to four hours. I didn't worry for Josh's safety, but I did worry our son would experience Jack's distress, or even worse, another attempt.

I had tried so hard to shield him from the drama through the years, but particularly from recent events. I called him and asked him to remain in his room until I could get home, and with no questions asked, he did.

The next day, flights resumed and Jack went to Dallas. The trip was uneventful, though Jack stressed his concerns about flying most of the way back to the airport. I had to dismiss his fears. I felt I had no other choice.

The next call I got was from his father, assuring me he had arrived safely.

Throughout Jack's stay in Dallas, I called daily, and he didn't sound well most days. His father and other family members expressed concerns about his stability. They called me every few days to tell me they feared he would take his life while living there unless he was with his family.

I sympathized.

No, I empathized. It was painful to hear their distress and I often wondered how I sounded on the other end of the phone to others listening from a distance. I reminded them he *had* been with us when he attempted to take his life the first time. He desperately needed treatment and I couldn't make that happen where we were. Yes, I empathized, but I felt we had no other earthly options.

Over the course of a few weeks, he settled in. We talked every day. If we had an agenda to discuss, then he could carry on a simple but effective conversation. If there was nothing of substance to discuss, we sank into dialogue about his condition and treatment. The conversation would then quickly digress into his begging and pleading to return home.

I had to be strong. The phrase "tough love," which I had so often said in sessions with clients, became a loud ringing in my ears every day. Much of what I taught and advised for my clients haunted my every moment. It was time to really walk the walk.

Jack didn't like his treatment. He didn't like his situation. He didn't like himself. And some days, he didn't like me, but I was certain he needed to stay there.

While the psychiatrist proved to be very eccentric and sometimes questionable in his practices, I encouraged Jack to continue going to treatment in Dallas. I saw no other option. I remember thinking I had truly become desperate for his survival.

10

THE RETURN HOME

JACK SUFFERED FROM REACTIONS to a number of medications. I suspected because he had never taken medications in his life, he was much more sensitive to them than most people, but maybe not.

Many people suffer negative effects from the medications used to treat mental health issues. The challenge is to find the right blend of medications to ease the symptoms and hopefully stabilize the person. The family takes the brunt of exaggerated symptoms brought on by medications that aren't the right match. It's so very frustrating many times there's just not a better way to treat mental illness except trial and error. And there are lots of errors.

We all grew weary of the process. Jack's tumultuous personality each and every day caused fatigue for everyone in his environment in Dallas. I was wearing thin from a distance. I began to promise if he just held on one more day, then all would be better. I begged him to hold on for his children or for me. The truth is, I really wanted him to do it for himself, but he couldn't. He had come to share the same ill regard for himself he felt others in his family had held for him all his life.

* * *

Jack landed a job in Dallas through the kindness of a close friend. Of course, it was a lesser position than he was accustomed to, but he was thankful at first.

When he told me about the job, I reflected back on his inability to "make sandwiches" at Subway a few months earlier. Thinking Subway would just be a "filler" position while he was in treatment, applied for a management position. Soon after he began, he came home in a fit of distress. He begged me to allow him to quit because he just couldn't remember how to make all the variations of sandwiches. It was too stressful for him.

His begging left me with an incredible sense of hopelessness. Jack's anxiety was unbearable to watch. I agreed he should quit, but I wondered whether it was actually the sandwich making or just that he just felt the job was beneath him.

I soon determined it was indeed the stress of sandwich making. He was losing the capacity to retain and process complex information—a character trait he had always prided himself on.

Despite my reservations about the Dallas job, I thought, "At least he has something to do."

After three weeks, I answered an unscheduled call.

"I need to return home," he announced. "No one likes me here. I have to get out of here!"

"What do you mean? Your family likes you. You need to stay in treatment until we find a better solution," I insisted.

Of course, the claim no one liked him was preposterous to me, but he was serious. His illness taught me to reframe my thoughts about absolutes.

"I need to go home now. Everyone is against me in this job. They are undermining me here," he pleaded.

I kept talking. Many times, regardless of the argument, my voice alone would calm him. I could only hope this would be the case this time. "Give me an example," I said.

I didn't know what to believe. Sometimes the business environment *is* brutal—dog-eat-dog, so to speak. This kind of tension drove him to success in previous years, but was it too rough for him now? I was tempted to believe his reaction was just paranoia. It was hard to tell these days. Sometimes he tried to draw me into his world of drama and chaos. Other days, he operated in the reality of the situation. I decided whether his fears were founded or not, it didn't matter. There was nothing else I could do this far away.

I couldn't see clearly anymore. I had become blinded by the illusion. The ability to push through to the other side of challenges had become a part of my character, but at what point does such a virtue become a flaw?

In July, Jack returned home from Dallas in time to help with the move to the new Tennessee city where I'd accepted the university position in February. Given the circumstances, we decided we'd all move together.

Our son was a junior in high school and I wanted to avoid moving him, but the option wasn't available. He was able to finish both his junior and senior years in the three months left before the move, quite a feat for a sixteen-year-old. Our son has his father's intellect and what I hope is my groundedness. He pushed through with honors.

As we prepared for the move, Jack seemed optimistic and encouraged by the new opportunity. He felt happy for me and expressed how proud he was at every turn. He also told me how grateful he was I had stayed with him. He became very emotional. He was thankful for what he had and very appreciative of me. It was nice.

While he was committed to the family now, but I had to grapple with the man he had become. It was heart wrenching to watch, but even more difficult to understand. Where had he gone? What happened to the man I married? I came to appreciate the phrase "Be careful for what you wish for, you just might get it."

The move went as smoothly as I could have imagined. I bought a house sight unseen in a city I had only been to twice in my life, once for the interview and once to take Josh to see the campus where I'd be teaching. Josh was so young when he finished high school, but he had been in a program in high school offering college credit. I felt like the university would be a placeholder until we got through the woods with his dad and he grew up some.

We looked at houses after the college tour, but I found nothing. I couldn't possibly return to look at homes. I needed to sell my business, finish up my consulting work, and assist our son with the transition.

I bought the house without seeing it because I wanted one thing to be known: where we would live. As much as I wanted to believe home is wherever your family is, there was too much instability in our family. Home became a stressful and unpredictable place. I was reminded this was what Jack knew growing up. It had been manifested for the rest of us now.

11

GREAT EXPECTATIONS

ONE WOULD EXPECT IN OUR NEW and larger city, getting into a clinic or getting an appointment to see a psychiatrist would have been easier. Again, it proved to be almost as difficult as our previous situation. Numerous offices were closed to new patients, and the ones that weren't had at least a two-week waiting period. I took an appointment and continued to look for a quicker solution.

Jack seemed much better during the day but deteriorated quickly in the evenings. It seemed like his prescriptions might just be wearing off by sunset. I didn't know whether that was true, but it was a pattern. In searching for answers, I asked Jack about what he was taking. The psychiatrist in Dallas recommended he open a Lithium capsule and pour it in water, drinking only a quarter of the solution per day. This seemed a bit archaic.

I later found out our health insurance didn't cover mental health medications either and this was a way Jack felt he could save money. The medication would have been several hundred dollars a month, but by doing it this way, the costs were significantly decreased. I felt that he wasn't getting what he needed and this method left a huge margin for error.

Also, the cost of seeing the psychiatrist for one week was as much his medications for the entire month. It was incredible! To this day I angrily question the logic of this physician. But then again, maybe this was just Jack's logic and justification, and the doctor had nothing to do with it. Either way, this was what he did until we found other solutions for his treatment.

In my desperation, I contacted a clinic in Atlanta that treated patients based on a brain scan. We traveled down to this clinic to find they didn't agree with his bipolar diagnosis and thought he had severe attention deficit hyperactivity disorder (ADHD). They had a more natural approach to treatment, so Jack gladly retreated from his medications. He was given a holistic treatment plan including supplements in lieu of harsh medications, exercise, and a nutrition plan.

Once he was off his medications, however, it was quite a challenge to get Jack to comply with his treatment regimen, and he progressively got worse. I understood the medications made him miserable and he didn't want to take them. Who would blame him? I didn't. I saw the wretched effects he had to contend with.

Since his experiences with liquid Lithium and the holistic care plan (which he refused to follow), the only treatment he received came from urgent care clinics when he was in distress. They changed his medications regularly because Jack could never find a solution to his pain, his anxiety, or panic attacks. They handed out medications like candy in these clinics, but they didn't provide any oversight for medication management or any follow-up, despite being the only places we could get him in regularly. It was incredible.

Throughout the year, there were times Jack seemed so collected and pulled together. When he was in his logical mind, all was well. But when he entered his emotional mind, he struggled.

This is why I believe so many psychiatric professionals thought he was okay. Initially, his symptoms didn't manifest until he tried to deal with his emotions. Matters of the heart were where he felt the least competent. He didn't know how to live from his heart, so it left him a defenseless child more and more often.

He began to read everything he could find on the subject of living a balanced life—one from the head *and* the heart. We would have intellectual conversations for hours about it. We would stay up discussing beliefs, spirituality, and the afterlife. He asked a lot of questions and shared his deepest thoughts. When I look back on it, anyone who heard our conversations might have thought it was crazy to be speaking about these things so rationally. I mostly lived and spoke from my heart more than my head but I had learned over the years to converse more analytically in order to communicate with Jack.

He frequently said things like, "I know I'm dying. What do you suppose it will be like?" and "When I die, I don't want to stay here. How can I move on to be with God?" and "What do you suppose it feels like to be free from illness and a body?"

I was comfortable with these conversations because I knew they helped him learn and grow into the man I knew was inside him. Ironically, in those days, he seemed to take up permanent residence in heart-based conversations and feel comfortable there.

It was when he had to be in his head, accessing knowledge and skills, science and math, he became stressed. The transition from who he had been to who he had become was remarkable. He didn't seem to be able to balance both the head and the heart of his being.

Daily, my emotions would swing from confidence he was on the right track to panic as I watched him crumple to the floor in despair. Emotions ran high each and every day. One moment he spoke like a scholar, and the next I consoled him as he sat crying on the floor of the kitchen. Days flew by and yet it felt as if we were caught in the folds of time with no way out. One minute we laughed together, the next he had death on his mind. It was almost debilitating for me, and my emotions wore thin. I needed some relief. I began to feel my own grip on reality slip.

Anxiety and panic attacks became a daily event for him; he had let go of the intellect and sense of humor he was known for—he just couldn't access them anymore. Desperation became more the norm than the exception. By the fall, the general feeling of the house had become morose and difficult to withstand. I felt compelled to call every day on my way home from the university so I'd have some idea what condition he would be in when I arrived. Despite the days of unmanaged desperation and anxiety, I still thought he would make it out of this.

Tense conversations in the kitchen became a daily ritual as the fear and anxiety began to rise in him in the latter part of each day. Regularly, he asked me to listen closely.

"You're tired, I'm tired. I'm done. I am in so much pain every day. I really think I have lung cancer now. My body is shutting down. I can feel it. I am nothing but a burden on you and the family. I can't bear to think about being a burden for the rest of my life. You need to help me push the reset button. I'll come back in and try this again."

"*No*, I won't say it's okay for you to leave us. You're just ill. You don't have cancer and I'm not going to help you do anything to leave."

I suspect the tone of my voice became more monotone and mocking over time. I hate to reflect back on this, but it was the truth. I became more and more dissociated from the situation to survive. I thought about the amazing people who are able to be present for years, caring for someone who is ill, mentally or otherwise. I wondered every day if I had the fortitude to do this.

There were days I felt ashamed I couldn't hold up under the onslaught. Surely there was help somewhere.

By September, Jack began cycles of starving himself, and even refusing to drink water, from Thursday through Tuesday. Why Thursday through Tuesday, I'm not entirely sure. I was home on the weekends so I thought he might do it to get my maximal attention for his hunger strikes.

I would go upstairs where he was sleeping and beg him to eat. He had already lost over sixty pounds in the last nine months due to stress and anxiety. He was wasting away. He also knew much about the physiology of the body and medicine. He knew going without food would never end his life, but it would only take four days for him to die of dehydration.

A deep exhaustion exacerbated my intolerance for drama and caused frequent moments of impatience. He would push himself. He would push me. I resented it and I told him so. I felt this vicious cycle was pure manipulation.

After three cycles, I couldn't be manipulated anymore. During his fourth attempt, I simply walked up the stairs on the third day and announced I would not ask him to eat or drink again. I demanded he get up and go to a hotel and die there. I could not have our son experience such a tragic death.

There was something about the feeling of being constantly manipulated I could not stand. I felt I had allowed myself to be manipulated long enough. This was not love; this was a little boy crying out for attention. When pressed, he agreed. He came down to eat dinner with us that evening.

In October, after he began constantly obsessing about taking his life and denied himself a sufficient amount of food to maintain his weight, his primary care physician admitted him to the hospital again, after a medication follow-up.

"Jack," he said, "I'm really worried. You seem to be in such distress, yet you're so calm and logical about it all. I don't feel comfortable with you going back home. There is a hospital nearby I want you to think about."

Jack responded, "Yeah, I guess it's time to give everyone a break."

What an odd response, I thought. I didn't care. Those words were such a relief to me.

I still had hope. Hope we would find the magic pill or the magic solution. It was critical he be seen in an intensive treatment environment. I also desperately needed a break. We were in the ninth month of distress. I felt him slipping away with every day, yet I couldn't find a solution. I thought if I could have a few days of sleep, I could focus on the solution.

We arrived at the hospital and I felt confident we were on the right path, though Jack was already showing signs of discontent with the facility when we arrived in the parking lot. He said the hospital looked like some boutique hotel. He questioned the competency of the staff.

"This place will just cost a lot of money," he argued.

Again, I ignored his concerns.

During his assessment, he admitted to trying to kill himself by starvation and declared he had no intention of remaining in the world. He was calm and resolved. He willingly gave me his wallet, his shoes with laces, and belt before he was asked. He knew the drill.

Jack called on his second day in the hospital.

"Can you come pick me up after noon today? I'm being discharged."

My heart sank. "No, you need to stay there longer. What have you done since you've been there?"

"Nothing!" he blurted out. "I've just stayed in my room. There was a social worker who came in a couple of times, and the physician consulted for five minutes. I told you, it'd be like staying in a hotel. I'm really bored and I want to be at home. I went to one session and we were drawing with crayons—ridiculous!"

He was discharged after two days. They told me they had to recertify patients with our insurance company every forty-eight hours, and it was too much work for a patient who truly wouldn't comply. I promptly called to talk with the psychiatrist on staff.

"We can't keep him. He doesn't want to participate in our group sessions. I'm not sure he belongs here anyway. He seems fully capable of handling this himself. This is a voluntary facility. He can leave when he wants to leave."

I was livid!

The day of discharge I called the family physician and said, "He can't leave! *Someone* has to help him. He's going to die at home if we don't do something. I need a counselor who can provide us with some guidance."

The counselor he referred us to was a breath of fresh air. She connected with me right away and was intelligent enough to keep up with Jack. She provided wonderful support for him over the coming days. But as competent as she was, she too had difficulty managing Jack's perspectives on life and death.

"I have never met anyone who could be so resolved and logical about taking his life." She said. "It makes therapy difficult because he doesn't seem to want to get better."

She worked with him twice a week. Later, she shared with me he told her the reason he'd agreed to meet with her was he knew I needed a break from his discussions about death. Though she felt she wasn't helpful, she will never know how much she helped him feel validated. That's what he needed: validation, and someone to just hold space for him to talk.

It seems to be such a small thing, but it's critical to feeling human. She was the first bright light in those dark days for both of us. She was the first mental health professional to demonstrate the compassion so critically needed in the care of people who are suffering.

12

BLURRED LINES

ONE MORNING, JACK VENTURED into the kitchen, while I made breakfast. "I had a dream that you will write a book," he said.

I laughed, "About what?"

"You'll write a book about our experiences. This book will help people heal." He went on, "I saw you writing this book about mental health challenges."

Again, I laughed. "I don't have the energy to write up my research, much less write a book."

"You will, I saw it," he assured me.

Life reverted to the way it had been before he was admitted to the hospital. He struggled to keep his composure each day. One day ran into the next with no break in drama or distress. We continued our long conversations in the evening, which now had become exhaustive Q & A sessions.

"What do you believe about people who choose to leave the earth voluntarily? Do you think they go to hell?" he asked.

"No," I would say, "but I believe the Creator of Life is about sustaining life. If someone chooses to end that life, I believe he or she will get a lesson or two about the value of life and living."

"*Mmmhmm.* Then there is no hell?" he said as he analyzed the situation.

"I don't believe in hell anymore," I said with a tired voice. "I believe we create our own circumstances by our choices. We are each here to learn valuable lessons so we become better people, better souls to honor God and humanity." Coming from a fearmongering background in the Southern Baptist church, I had come a long way to be able to confess my convictions about hell. "I believe God is everywhere and everything is God. Evil in the world is manifested by the negative choices we make that are not in alignment with the goodness of God," I continued.

The tenor of these conversations became calmer over the course of the next few weeks, and it felt more like he was a student asking important and relevant questions in class. When we talked, he was calm, connected, and attentive. He had a sense of peace about him. For me, there were glimmers of hope in each of these conversations, as morbid as they may have seemed to an outsider. He was finding himself in them.

And yet, days when we didn't have those conversations, he cycled into the chasm of despair. In the first week of November, he pleaded with me again, "*Please* help me find a way to do this gently. I can't bear the pain of you or our sons thinking I suffered."

"No, I'm sorry, Jack, I can't do that. We want you here. I want to share grandchildren with you one day."

His affect became grave. The drama escalated from that day forward.

My family decided to come for Thanksgiving and I called to let them know things weren't good. Besides, I didn't know if I was up to company, as wonderful as it would be to see them. I was tired and I didn't see this ending any time soon. I put my family's plans on hold, pending Jack's condition leading up to their trip. In the meantime, Jack and I had an anniversary coming and I had no idea what to do. I continued to go through the motions at work to stay afloat. I taught a relatively heavy schedule and worried about when I would have the time or energy to write up my research.

I was still fully committed to Jack's recovery... but doubts crept in. What if it never came? What would I do if he never got better? I hadn't considered that until now, but clearly it was a possibility.

Late one evening after an exhausting, frenetic discussion, I escaped to the bathroom. Balancing on the edge of the bath, I began to cry. The realization I could not save him sank in. I realized in that moment he was waiting on me to let him go. I had been opposing him for so long now I couldn't see the obvious. I had to let go of him.

I just couldn't, not yet. What if he chose to go? Could I live with myself?

"What if I allow him his freedom and he decided not to fight?" I thought.

His mortality was not for me to dictate. I loved him and I watched him suffer every day. I decided the most loving thing I could possibly do for him was to honor his wishes. I had to give him the freedom he'd been begging for since last February.

In so many ways, I felt like a hypocrite. I counseled clients about unconditional love and loving detachment, but I was still attached to the outcomes of his decisions. I was angry he would put me in this position. I was frustrated and scared.

Soon, a calmness I couldn't explain came over me. Indeed, I had to let go of the outcome of all of this. I finally sank down to the floor and cried tears of relief. I felt peace that defied all understanding—especially my own. I slept well that night.

* * *

The next morning, I rose early. When the sun peeked over the horizon, rays of sunshine burst in through the high ceiling windows in the living room. The light was particularly harsh this morning and I moved to the dining room. I dropping down onto the same unforgiving dining room chair I had centered in the room months ago to protect Jack from hurting himself after his first attempt. I wearily leaned over the card I purchased for our upcoming anniversary. I reflected on how difficult it had been to select an appropriate card this year, how I, an otherwise decisive person, could be reduced to loitering in a gift store for an hour, struggling to choose a card.

It had come to this. No card could express the depths with which I had come to know Jack and the feeling he was rapidly slipping away. No card could reflect the unconditional commitment I felt, yet the morbid idea I was letting go.

My hand trembled. As I look back on that day, I still don't know if the tremble was from exhaustion, sadness, or purely resolution. My message to him began:

"Jack, I give you your freedom."

I knew I had to let him go, but how? With my deep convictions about the sanctity of life and living, I struggled hard to let go. It was as if I were condoning his decision, his behavior. My deep Southern Baptist beliefs bubbled up and stared me in the face a number of times that morning. But fear and judgment had to give way to love and compassion.

I cried tears of profound sadness, anger, joy—and relief.

* * *

Later that morning, I gave him the card in the kitchen.

"Happy anniversary," I whispered. "I want you to know I love you and always will. I can let you decide now what your soul needs to be happy."

All I could hear was my heart beating out of my chest. Then a deafening silence rushed into the room.

He read the card, standing as quiet and as motionless as someone in the woods when there's a natural predator rambling through. First, a look of shock came over his face, and then it softened to one of relief.

He looked at me with tears in his eyes. "Thank you so much. This is an incredible gift. I know how hard this must have been for you. I have loved you all of my life and I know I'm killing you. You know this is the right thing to do."

I stared at him in disbelief.

A part of me had expected him to say, "I can't believe you would give me a card like this!" or maybe "You're abandoning me."

Or even better, "You know I can't really carry through with this."

That didn't happen. I felt like God was calling my bluff about unconditional love and commitment. There was no turning back now. As much as I wanted to retract my offer, I couldn't. It was out there. It read:

Jack, I give you your freedom.

While all of this seems so surreal, I do know and understand that you are done with this life. I also understand that there is nothing more I can do to keep you in this world. I too now feel at peace with whatever you decide is right for you. As we experience the 19th year of marriage, I have only one gift to give you now... your freedom. Whatever this means, wherever you go, please remember that we have always loved you, will always remember you, and you will always be with us.

I cannot begin to understand the pain you feel and the longing you have to leave. What I can understand is that it's a pain so deep that you need relief. I know you have always loved us in the best way you knew how to love. It was enough.

I hope you find "enough" wherever you are. You have blessed my life in a way you'll never know.

Happy Anniversary,
Me

* * *

I called my family and they gladly drove in for Thanksgiving. At this point, I knew there might be little time. They understood the gravity of the situation and respectfully and lovingly engaged Jack in as much normalcy as they could muster.

Jack didn't join us for the activities of the day. Despite it being painful for us all, he insisted he not sit at the table with us for the Thanksgiving meal. He sat lonely at the bar on a wobbly stool with a base that had needed tightening for a year. As had become typical, he sat picking at his food, moving it around from one side of the plate to the other, like the boys would do as children when they wanted me to believe they'd taken several bites.

Having a low tolerance for drama, I fought my instinct to call him out on this foolishness, but I didn't. I let him have his drama. I let him have control. He'd felt so out of control for so long. He didn't see he'd had his family by the neck, controlling our every move, for almost three years.

It was so hard to allow him to do what he needed to do. I wanted to be gentle, but my gentleness felt depleted. I wanted to be kind, but I felt exploited. I really wanted to scream *"Stop it!"* from a mountaintop so there was no doubt that he could hear me.

He sat on that stool, reminding me in a big way he was going, and not even granting us the kindness of sitting with us at the table. He withdrew slowly, carving himself out of the family. Everyone felt guilty. His depression hung like a heavy cloud over the holiday.

He maintained his composure through the visit and I knew he was doing it for me. He retreated to his office upstairs, where he could lie down, often and for progressively longer periods of time. It felt as if he was grieving. Grieving where he was in life. Grieving his own loss and what he was about to lose.

My frequent visits to his locked door were unproductive and felt almost intrusive. Sometimes he responded with a muffled "No thank you" and other times he didn't answer at all.

By the third night, my brother, Sam, convinced him to go out and have a holiday drink with him. While they were out, Jack asked him to take care of us. They had a long, serious conversation that left Sam completely disarmed. Later that evening, Sam asked me to sit down at the dining room table.

"He's really not well," he said.

I hadn't seen my brother cry since he was eight years old but tears of frustration and agony ran down his cheeks. Sam lost an old roommate and best friend to suicide a few years prior to this.

"I saw this in Seth." He said. "He was bipolar and it progressed exactly this."

He told me about the conversations he and Seth had. I listened intently. They were the same conversations Jack and I had so logically each night in the kitchen.

Had I lost my mind? The danger, the distress, the panic in Sam's voice scared me a bit. He confronted me with such honesty; I didn't know what to say.

"He has to be admitted soon. He has to be admitted to a long-term treatment facility," he stressed. "He is not well. This isn't good."

I didn't tell him about the anniversary card. I was ashamed to tell him I'd given Jack his freedom. Maybe I just wasn't strong enough and had given up. I didn't know.

The conversation with my brother was the first time someone told me what to do. Not one of the psychiatrist or psychologists we'd seen had a clue what to do with Jack. This was the first time I could recall being given what I believed to be a real solution. Why hadn't I thought of a long-term treatment facility?

Quite honestly, up until the last week, I may have been in denial he was that sick. A strange duality had existed for quite some time. I was convinced he would heal or we'd find a solution right around the corner. The optimist in me won out over and over. Maybe just around the next corner... but it just was never there. There was a tree and a tree and a tree, but I couldn't see the forest.

A long-term treatment facility. *Yes!* I could do that. It seemed so logical. I could find a facility that could help him. If he stayed long enough, they'd have to discover what was wrong. Though it was a Saturday evening, I promptly called his psychologist.

She answered. She said she had come to the same conclusion and had already suggested this plan to Jack during his last session. Though thrilled to have a consensus, I was somewhat deflated knowing he had chosen not to tell me. Regardless, I pressed forward. This was the key to the puzzle. He couldn't outwit them all if he had to stay a month or even three months. I sat down at my computer, all holiday celebrations coming to a halt.

As I searched for facilities, I began to understand why this option had not been raised before. I found many of these facilities were not covered by our insurance. The insurance coverage we had at the university was among the best available, yet the facilities our insurance covered were short-term or state mental facilities. The first option hadn't been successful and the latter wasn't available in our state.

With no regard for cost, I searched deep into the night. By the next day I narrowed it down to three possible facilities. The last and potentially most prohibitive piece of the puzzle was how to fund his stay. These facilities were $5,000 to $15,000 a month.

I was convinced I could find the money somewhere.

We went to see the psychologist the following Tuesday to discuss options. Jack thought we were still discussing short term or outpatient care. He wasn't aware of my conversation with the therapist about long term care.

Before we left for the appointment, I overheard Jack, who sat with our son on the edge of the worn leather couch. It was relatively new, but this was the couch Jack slept on for hours each day, whenever he needed to escape his anxiety, was adjusting to a new medication, or was simply too tired to move.

Passing through, all I heard of this conversation was the phrase "I promise you I won't harm myself. We're going to make this work."

Those were the first words of encouragement I had heard from him in months. Turning the corner, I gave a deep sigh of relief. The man I had married, while he may have been disconnected, was honest. He would never make a promise he couldn't keep. If there was one trait I really admired in Jack, it was his honesty about what he was willing and not willing to do. This was good news!

Contemplating how to best present the idea of a long-term care facility, I followed him to the therapist's office. He insisted on driving to the appointment separately, which was unusual because his anxiety had kept him from driving any distance for 3 months at this point. Jack parked swiftly and abruptly jumped from his vehicle as if he were dodging a wasp. He scuffled quickly inside, head down with no eye contact with any one. He was nervous and obviously tense.

I sat down alongside him on the bench in front of his therapist's office and waited. The tension in the hallway was electric. Though I hadn't shared the plan with him, he sat rigid and uncomfortable on the bench as if he were a child waiting for vaccinations at the doctor's office. It was as if he intuited what he was about to face.

During the counseling session, he began to waffle. He became very agitated and distressed as we presented the option of a long-term facility. I knew this would be hard for both of us but it felt like a good option. He tried to leave the session a couple of times and he expressed concerns about being away from his family for that long.

He kept saying, "I won't live away from my family. I just won't survive." The irony of that statement told me he wasn't as resolved about dying as he professed.

We talked about other options for treatment and the fact we would visit any chance we got. He left the session in palpable distress. I worried about his safety but he was gone when I got to the parking lot. That evening, he wanted nothing to do with the conversation. He went directly to what had become his room and closed and locked the door. I continued to search for options that night. I just knew we were onto something.

The next day, he seemed calmer, but he'd reverted back to cycles of logic and distress by the evening hours. I tried to gently introduce the idea of moving to an area that had a treatment facility, but we exchanged few words at a time about this subject.

Finally, the root of his distress came out. "I will never leave a place like that. I know this in my heart. I will be admitted and will never get out."

All the reassuring in the world wasn't going to convince him otherwise. He felt stripped of his manhood, and all the things he feared most were coming to fruition, particularly his fear of abandonment. I grieved for him but knew we had to find a solution for us all. Time was of the essence now.

By Thursday, the sun seemed to fill the house again. There were mornings when I relished the beauty of the sun shattering the darkness. Other days, I resented it. It was so out of reach. I could see it but I couldn't experience it. I couldn't enjoy it, so I didn't want it.

I arose and found him already making breakfast in the kitchen. Shocked, I remarked, "Well, this is a nice surprise! You must be feeling good today." I started asking the usual questions in search of the source of this positive affect. I asked, "How did you sleep? Have you taken your medications?"

"Yes!" he said, almost shattering the tranquility of the moment. It was almost as if he didn't want any threats to his positive attitude.

Feeling doubtful, I quickly recovered. "Okay, well... you just seem different. You're much more like yourself this morning. I was just curious what may be different."

He continued whistling and preparing breakfast. The change was remarkable. I hadn't heard him whistle in more than a year. Desperate for a solution, as well as having a researcher's mentality, I wanted to know what was and wasn't working. The last three years had been devastating, and now, overnight, all was well?

While I was curious about this change, I was happy about it and decided to leave it alone for the time being. I actually felt relief, a feeling I hadn't had in months. Not the same relief I felt when I conceded about his future, but relieved that maybe we were turning the corner.

"Have you decided to try the long-term treatment?" I asked.

He replied in almost a singsong tone, "It will all be okay. I've got it handled. I'm working out the details now. You need to relax... and don't worry so much. I know how tired you are. No worries for you today, my dear!"

Hesitantly, I smiled, agreed, and left the room to get ready for work. My mind explored what options he could be researching. We had also discussed temporarily moving to a nearby suburb that had an outpatient program.

"Maybe he's checking into that option," I thought. "Yes, that would be so great!"

13

THE BEGINNING

I HAD SUCH A GOOD DAY at work. After having a good morning with Jack, I felt hope creeping back into the equation. The only thoughts about him that came to my mind during the day were optimistic ones. I was relieved he felt better and didn't think any further than that. Worry had been a faithful friend over the last several months and that day I felt better than I had in a long, long time.

I left work in the afternoon. The sun shone and it seemed the air was lighter, friendlier. I found myself humming to music in the car and enjoying the ride home. I thought about what we could have for dinner. I wondered if he might even feel like eating that night. He was down almost seventy pounds from a normal, healthy weight. So obviously, he could use some calories.

My friend Mary called to check on us and I actually felt like talking. She encouraged me again to visit her in Mexico, where she lived several months of the year. Part of me wanted to book the flight right away.

I arrived at the house and saw Jack's car in the driveway. Though Jack wasn't driving much anymore, it brought my thoughts to him. A flicker of concern crept over me, but I washed it away as I laughed with my friend on the phone. Friends and family consciously made an effort to make me laugh. Some days I feigned laughter or mustered a chuckle, because most days, humor was not a part of my life. To truly laugh was a remarkable change.

I parked in the garage and climbed the stairs. As I entered the house, everything smelled fresh, as if it had been cleaned. And it had. The floors were mopped and the kitchen tidied. Sun shone through crystal clear windows, glinting on the freshly cleaned cabinets. As I talked with Mary, I looked around. Dinner simmered on the stove. The coffeepot stood ready, prepared for the next day. When he was well, Jack had always made my coffee, something I missed after he'd become ill.

I entered the bedroom to take off my shoes and began to get comfortable. Everything I saw reinforced my feeling Jack must have had a good day. Everything was in order, with the comforter smoothed, the pillows plumped. It was as if I'd had a housekeeper come in.

We'd spent the last three years living through one of Jack's "downs," but the current state of the house reminded me of the time before he lost his job, when he seemed to be flourishing as he attempted to step into the family circle. He had been good about helping around the house then. I appreciated it so much because his housekeeping was much better than mine. I tended to do a global cleaning, but he paid attention to the details. I never liked cleaning baseboards or cracks and crevices. He did. He was meticulous.

I said goodbye to Mary and hung up the phone. I called out to Jack, anxious to thank him for doing such a wonderful job on the kitchen.

No answer.

I climbed the stairs, thinking he may have been taking a nap. The door to his office was closed. Not unusual.

But there was something out of sorts. A note leaned against the door. *How did he get that to lean against a closed door like that?* I thought.

I froze.

I stared at the note. I could read it from where I stood, but it seemed to move farther and farther from me. "My Darling," it said.

I stood with no breath left. I took in air at a rapid rate to keep from blacking out. I couldn't breathe. The room siphoned all the oxygen away from my brain.

I couldn't process what I saw. I felt like I was attempting to do one of those exercises in kindergarten—"What doesn't belong?" A deep disconnect plunged between this moment and the earlier happenings of the day.

As I stood there, a sense of dread overwhelmed me. It seemed like everything was underwater and moving in slow motion as I picked up the letter with trepidation.

Each time I began to read the words, I would have to reread them. I couldn't process them.

It said, "My Darling, do not open the door. Let someone else take care of me. You should go call someone now who will take care of everything."

I couldn't comprehend the message. I read it again as tears began to well in my eyes. I don't recall breathing. A high-pitched noise buzzed in my head so loud I could barely hear myself pounding on the locked door.

"Don't lock me out!" I screamed. "Don't leave me!"

Nothing happened.

Part of me expected him to open the door right away, but he'd locked me out of his world, again, like he had done so many times before.

The commanding voice I now recognized as my own emerged. "Open the door! Open the door! Open the door!"

I gathered my wits and repeated to myself, "Don't go in... call someone." *Who do I call?*

I couldn't think. There was a surreal drag in time. I stood staring at the door, but I wasn't forming a plan for what to do.

I staggered down the stairs, measuring each step carefully in case I fainted. I found my phone and I called 911. I called and I couldn't speak. It was as if someone had tied my vocal cords in a knot.

"My..." I cleared my throat. "My husband is locked in a room. He left a note to call and it said not to enter the room. I'm afraid he's gone."

I couldn't comprehend anything but the 911 operator's directions to listen for an ambulance siren. And I did. I listened.

The siren began wailing from what seemed to be miles and miles away. It grew closer and closer. I stood at the front door, watching and waiting. I tried to remember why I was standing there. Shock consumed me, dragging me down into an abyss. I shivered violently.

No tears—just a body out of control. My brain told me to move away from the door when the paramedics arrived. I stood aside, suspended in time, while they rushed in and up the stairs.

There were many of them. Police cars arrived. I collapsed in a chair by the stairs.

I began to cry uncontrollably as they broke down the door, loud cracks of wood reverberating through the house. Deep pain throbbed through my solar plexus.

At that moment, I felt him. I felt him in a way that told me he was gone. I felt him wrap his arms around me from the back like he would sometimes when something good happened in his life, and I calmed. My body felt a cathartic release of pain, fatigue, and sorrow.

A voice murmured above me. I looked up into the teary eyes of a paramedic. I made out the words through the buzzing in my ears.

"Your husband is gone, I'm so sorry, ma'am. He was gone hours ago."

Numbness crept over me. It helped me get through all of the questions and chaos. More people arrived, police, detectives, support personnel. They gave me cards and numbers to call.

My head hurt. I felt as if I could sleep for days and then maybe this nightmare would be over.

They were all very helpful, but my brain could not fathom the reality of what had just happened, much less numbers and instructions.

I began to come around to what was most important now: the living. "My son!" My mind raced. *Where was Josh?*

I searched my brain for the answer. "He's at work." I relaxed, relieved he would not walk in on such a horrific scene. "Thank you, God."

After several moments, a police officer approached me. "Ma'am," he said. "Go to your room. We're bringing him down. I don't think you should be here."

He was right. I couldn't bear to see Jack—not now and not like this.

I retreated to my room. The walls seemed to move gently. I could feel the very spin of the Earth. I climbed up onto what had been my own bed for years. I lay in a loose fetal position and I cried. I closed my eyes and tears dripped from the corners.

This night didn't feel violent. It didn't feel like the grand crescendo of someone's dramatic life. It felt like a soft departure, a dignified fading out.

I felt loved in that moment; I felt Jack there, ever so slightly spooning me on the bed. I had the same feeling one might have after a long theatrical masterpiece, exhausted but longing for more.

Part of me was relieved it was over; part of me struggled with the void.

"It is done," a voice whispered in my head. The phrase reverberated in my mind as a reflection of my religious upbringing, but it signified the conclusion of this long-fought battle.

* * *

The detective quietly rapped on my door. "Do you have family in the area who I can call?"

I whispered through the thickness of the moment, "No, I don't, but I'll be okay. I just need to lay here for a while. Thank you."

I assured him I would be okay. I needed to be alone. I just needed to *feel.* I realized the act of feeling hadn't been an option for quite some time.

Despite the chaos, I felt calmer than I ever imagined I could feel under those circumstances. Was it shock? Or maybe it was the realization God had charge of Jack now.

I was off duty. Or I'd been relieved of my duties. And what a relief. I had felt sorely inadequate for the task of keeping the man alive any longer.

* * *

The room faded in and out of focus as I thought about the last few days.

A cleft in the heavy, light-blocking red curtains on my wall exposed the sliver of a waxing day-old moon. The cusps were sharp and defined. My mother always called it "God's fingernail."

Many nights when the boys were young, we gazed upon a waxing or waning moon to find the sharp cusps, talking about their grandma and the many phrases she'd passed down to me.

The moon and I were longtime lovers, and I knew this moon meant new beginnings. But how could I possibly begin again? "I don't have the energy," I thought.

The moon created a space of protection and love. I felt my body sinking deeply into the mattress and into a state of paralysis as I watched the moon flicker. I lay in unconscious dialogue with the moon.

I realized the moon represented so much more than what I could comprehend in that moment. There were days when the moon was gentle and loving, like the mother energy many cultures profess it to be; other days it felt like we were hanging on her very cusp, dangling helplessly over a vast, relentless sea of hopelessness.

* * *

After a while, my whole body jolted awake. I looked around at the dark room. What was I supposed to do next? Who should I call?

I sat down and cried for a moment—actually for several moments. In those quiet minutes, as I sobbed, I felt Jack's presence again, his body light and liberated. He assured me it would be okay. "This is clearly a new beginning for us both," he said.

* * *

I texted our son and told him to come right home after work. He told me later he knew by that text Dad was gone.

* * *

The next day, among all of the many things I had to do, I learned Nelson Mandela had died the same day as Jack. It was meaningful to me. Jack was in very good company.

14

CIRCLE OF LOVE

AS THE DAYS PASSED, I found more and more evidence Jack had been planning this for quite some time. The clean house and dinner preparation were only the beginning. He organized tax information for the coming year, and left explicit instructions for me. He paid bills in advance. He canceled credit cards and used up all of his checks with no reorder. He closed his email account and deleted his Facebook page.

He even discarded his carved pumpkin. Every year, I got one for each of us to carve. His pumpkin rarely got carved, but this year it had. I hadn't gotten around to disposing of them. I wish I had. Josh's, David's, and mine sat in a family on the porch. Jack's was gone.

He removed all pictures of himself from the frames around the house, giving an emotional respite to all who entered. For months he slowly culled and donated his belongings so they were all gone by the end. It was akin to the nesting a mother goes through before the birth of her child, but in reverse.

It was beautiful and considerate and loving, but he had erased all evidence of his existence from our surroundings. Knowing the police would confiscate his computer and any personal belongings, he left clear instructions on the desktop of his computer, outlining what he wanted to be done with his remains for the detective.

He'd thought of everything.

For days, I found boxes of my favorite movie candy hidden around the house—in places where only I would find them. I found sixteen boxes of candy.

He had clearly and carefully executed his plan. He had just been waiting on me to give him freedom, and that's all it took.

A week after his death, I found a long, beautiful letter from him tucked away. He hid this second letter because he knew the police would take the letter he'd left at his office door as evidence.

It was a love letter. A love letter like he'd never written before. A love letter from a place of remarkable unselfishness.

Love letters so often describe how someone can't live without someone else or what one will do if his or her needs don't get met. This love letter wasn't about Jack at all; it was about me, and the boys. He wanted us to be okay, and he wanted us to begin again with no attachments. He went on to say he knew he and his illness would be a burden to us. He said he knew solutions were hard to come by for people like him.

He included my anniversary card, clearly reminding me I had been a willing participant in his decision by giving him his freedom.

When I found the letter, my knees gave way. Part of me was so full of love and grateful to have this letter, and part of me cursed him under my breath.

* * *

I hesitated to share his letter because it's so personal, but vulnerability makes us more human. Jack learned so many beautiful lessons in his journey. I would be remiss not to share them.

Part of the letter read:

Just as it's impossible for me to know how I have blessed your life, so too is it difficult for me to completely convey the messages you have carried to me. These are things I know are the true meaning and purpose of a life embraced:

- *Everything is about people, connection, and love.*

- *There is no greater reward than learning through service to others.*

- *No matter how hard one works to keep things "perfect," it is impossible to achieve such a state of living.*

- *Life is supposed to be a challenge so that we may reach beyond ourselves.*

- *Genuine appreciation for what we have, such as kindness, tenderness, selflessness,*

- *Awareness of the miracles that surround us... being able to really experience these*

- *Without the interference of the reality that there is no guarantee of a specific outcome... or even tomorrow.*

- *The more we seek to understand others, the more we discover the Universe.*

- *We must bravely accept what God has placed before us.*

- *There is no such thing as control over the outside world. We experience control only over ourselves... how we act, react, think and behave toward others.*

- *I believe the greatest achievement for each of us is to be able to respond to all outside forces with integrity, honesty, self-assurance, compassion, empathy, and without fear. At the root of fearlessness is the state of knowing that all will be okay and as it should be.*

As hard as it was to receive his letter, it was a deep lesson for me. If he learned so much, then why couldn't he embrace this for his life ahead? After reading this, I knew in my heart he was truly done.

For weeks to come, I saw him everywhere. I heard him in so many songs that played. I understood from my work this was a normal grief response, but strange happenings seemed to be suspiciously timed in ways that brought tears to me and others around me. Family and friends felt what I felt: he was incredibly close, each and every day. It was comforting, yet frustrating.

Many times, I would wake in the middle of the night, though it seemed like I had just fallen asleep. I wanted so badly to see him in my dreams, but I just couldn't get to a dream state before abruptly waking, losing all opportunity to see him again.

In one of the many conversations we had, he told me he would come in my dreams so I would know he was okay. It wasn't until he was gone three months I finally had a dream about him.

He was healthy and happy. His face glowed with love and joy. He had brought messages, keys to healing, as he said he would.

15

CLOSURE

JACK WOULD BE SURPRISED by the impact his death had on people. Near the end, he became obsessed with the idea he had no friends, concerned he'd not spent the time developing relationships. While this was mostly true, after his death, the number of people who came forward to share the impact Jack had on their lives was remarkable. Most of these were people he had met in the last five years, when he was finally opening up to the heart.

He was such an enigma. I used to tell him 20 percent of his behavior affected 80 percent of his human beauty. We all have qualities that cause us to stumble. We're all here to learn.

Why Jack became the man he became is a mystery. Was it because he had a mental health issue left untreated all of his life? Was it the neglect he felt in his upbringing? Did something snap in his brain because he had a brilliant mind that saw the world in a very different way than most?

Does it really matter?

At this point, we can only take the moments and make them memories—memories that define us. These moments, good and bad, make us who we are. I cherish the last year of his life for this reason. It truly was a gift. I may have felt each day I couldn't make it through one more, but we had time together. We made memories for a lifetime. We shared a love that flowed deep into our souls and changed us both.

Most importantly, I believe he was happy with his decision. He truly believed he needed some work and he would come back in and start over.

For the living, the healing process is not to be ignored. We are the ones left behind. When tragedies like this one occur, we spend our time reaching for answers about why they happened or what we could have done differently.

If we love unconditionally, then we accept even when we don't understand or maybe even don't agree. We must let go of the things we cannot control and focus on what we can. It's part of the journey to wholeness.

16

THE JOURNEY BACK

HEALING FROM A LOSS TO SUICIDE seems different than from other losses. Not worse. Just different.

In a way, Jack's action insulted our family, making us feel we weren't important enough for him to live. The assurances he gave Josh two days before he died, that he would never hurt himself, felt like a slap in the face.

Exhaustion forced a numbness on me that somehow felt cathartic, but I also felt like I'd lost. It wasn't driven by ego or competition. I felt I'd lost to illness. I'd lost to death and ultimately lost the life my kids and I had known.

I'm not sure any of us is completely prepared to lose a loved one even when it's inevitable. The human spirit thrives on hope.

While hope is our best friend in times of need, lingering glimmers of hope may keep us hanging on emotionally until the last breath.

As I embarked on the journey to healing, it felt like it had been a very long trip already. I would have liked to treat this experience like the military relationships I had as a child, where I just moved past them quickly and easily, and rarely look back. But an event like this one deserved my full attention, so I could heal in a way that wasn't just "moving past" but immersing myself in the pain so it became real.

* * *

The days following Jack's death are hard to remember. I felt like I was helplessly floating face down in a vast dark ocean. It was peacefully frightening.

I had to push forward. There is so much to do following a death and I didn't feel like doing any of it. It was required and necessary, yet no one told me how to proceed.

When the first responders arrived, they tried to give me information, but I was in no frame of mind to retain it. It was as if Charlie Brown's teacher were talking. I heard voices but couldn't really make out the words.

In retrospect, it would have been so helpful if the first responders left a checklist of things I needed to do in the coming days, weeks, and months. I'm sure someone has thought about this and it's available somewhere, but I was alone in a new city with no idea how to proceed.

Jack's death came during final exams week at the university. I was not emotionally or mentally available for much else, yet I had to be. Life does not stop for the weary. All of us have responsibilities and those don't go away when you lose someone.

In the early stages of loss, one might argue this is by design. When tragedy strikes, it's as if the brain needs time to rest before processing what just happened, so the body stays busy, exerting as much energy as possible.

I stayed very busy. My body needed to stay in constant motion so I could not process the gravity of what had happened until I completed all the work ahead.

Early on, one person after another commented how well I was doing, and while I appreciated the acknowledgment, I wasn't doing well. For me those comments were clear indicators I *wasn't* well. I wasn't allowing the healing to come. I wasn't *feeling* the pain.

Actually, it was more of the same behaviors I'd used to cope with the ongoing stress of Jack and his illness. I was compartmentalizing my emotions to survive until the next moment. I was doing what I'd always done and what many people do to push through. But pushing through wasn't going to cut it this time. There was always going to be a gash in my being that could be seen deep in my falsely happy eyes if one looked close enough.

When Jack died, I experienced more compassion than I ever had, but also more judgment. Moving through his death was hard enough without the deep-rooted stigma of suicide in the Bible

Belt South. I wasn't prepared to address the uncomfortable questions about Jack's death.

I received a message from a longtime work friend who wrote it was so unfortunate to lose such a great guy to hell.

I wanted to unleash all my pent-up emotions on her, but I didn't. I recognized she didn't know what to say about the loss of a loved one. She hadn't acquired the resources to be tactful.

I just replied, "Thank you for recognizing he was a great guy, I believe he's experiencing love, peace and joy. I don't think those qualities exist in what you call hell."

* * *

Four weeks after his death, I opted to take a vacation to Mexico to see Mary. Jack actually insisted I take it the day before he died. I needed to go. I needed to go for a number of reasons. It gave me a refuge where I could think and process what had just happened. After the first day, I couldn't cry again. My tears were dammed up inside. I felt if I abruptly dropped the floodgates, it would destroy any semblance of life ahead of me. I held steady until God could work magic.

The first gift I received was the lesson nothing ever stays the same. As I began to plan the trip, I found myself holding my breath as I realized where Mary lived on the Mexican coast. It was forty-five minutes from Cozumel; the place Jack had taken me for our honeymoon nearly twenty years before, where we dove in the magnificent Caribbean. Mary and I spent two days on the island, hoping to reclaim those gentle, beautiful memories. It seemed I had so few good ones left. I needed those.

But nothing was the same. Tortuga was gone. It was as if my entire remembrance of what was had been absorbed in the folds of time. I felt a deep sense of loss. I questioned my memory. Had I made up the experiences I remembered? I didn't think so, but I recognized absolutely nothing.

Mary and I returned to Akumal, where she lived part-time. The next day, it took everything in my being to motivate my body to move. Mary, an expert diver, suggested we go to the community beach to snorkel. The sea turtles were active this time of year. I agreed.

My rational mind overtook my body's screaming to stay in bed. I knew I would regret missing a swim with the turtles. Besides, the turtle has always been my totem. At the risk of being accused of cultural appropriation, my grandmother was Choctaw and my family from Southeastern Oklahoma. My father also documented genealogy connecting us back to the "animal speakers" in the Druid culture in Scotland. I've always been drawn to all things of nature.

The beautiful beaches of Akumal were therapeutic yet frightening. I felt frail and vulnerable in this new place. That feeling was foreign to me. Traveling had always represented adventure to a military kid.

At our diving site, appropriately titled Turtle Bay, giant sea turtles hatched their eggs on the beach and made the calm emerald and turquoise waters their home. It felt safe and, at the time, I knew I needed safety.

Trauma had consumed my life, rendering me almost nonfunctional. I didn't feel unrecoverable, but it was paralyzing in the moment. I thought this must be what it felt like to face a giant black bear on a mountain trail. But it was more like being a trapped bird; appearing illogically calm when in reality it's immobilized by excruciating fear. I was exactly like that. I feared any movement would only cause more damage.

Floating on the ocean's surface with foggy goggles, I thought about the times Jack and I were in the ocean. He was an experienced dive master, and he and I dove together many times—including during our trip to Mexico. If my mask fogged, he'd remove it and spit in it, rub it, rinse it, and refit it to my face. Diving was the one time I felt he took care of me.

Scuba diving is very technical and my brain is not. Swimming on a swim team in Okinawa as a child made me comfortable in the water, but only when I was on the surface. In this moment, just floating on top with a snorkel felt overwhelming.

I just let my mask fog. Fog is exactly what my life was—a paralyzing fog. I smiled weakly at each passing turtle shadow, but only saw a hazy representation of the creatures. I gladly accepted a less-than-perfect view—a metaphor for my life at the time, I'm sure. I was accustomed to accepting what was rather than pushing toward what could or should be.

As Jack's paranoia and anxiety had mounted, I had to live day to day, and not because I was "living consciously," as I so often told myself; I was merely surviving. There was too much at stake to imagine a future. Staying shortsighted made me feel like my life was controllable, even when it wasn't.

Hypnotized by the rocking of gentle waves, I became lost in a sea of emotion. At first, I thought my mask might have been leaking, but the water on my cheeks felt warmer than the ocean around me. I realized tears bathed my face. It had been almost a month since Jack had taken his life and I could finally cry.

Underwater, tears dropped into my mask as a cathartic moan emerged from my chest. Shocked by it myself, I looked around for the movement of people underwater to see if anyone else had heard me.

Mindlessly, I paddled my feet, almost forgetting where I was, forgetting what I was doing—almost forgetting to breathe. Salty tears cleared the fog from my mask. As I relaxed, the brilliant colors came alive.

I turned to take in the newfound beauty of the undersea world and caught a shadow in the corner of my eye. A giant black eel abruptly charged my face! The viciousness of his smile and the black snakelike body startled me awake. A gurgling scream came from the water as I attempted a full reverse. Familiar fear raced through my body. I felt assaulted but strangely aware.

Fear of the unknown paralyzed me and, ironically, fear of the unknown awakened me. Though I didn't recognize it at the time, I think my healing began that day.

* * *

I returned home feeling a deep-cutting void. The frigid air bit my fingers as I put my bags in the trunk in long-term parking at the airport. I climbed into the car, dropping into the driver's seat. Stabilized by the steering wheel, I allowed the floodgates to open. I cried what seemed a lifetime of tears.

A small voice in the back of my mind startled me into awareness. "Nothing ever stays the same. Move forward. There's no going back now. Healing comes only when you are living in the moment."

I knew it was true, but it made me angry.

* * *

I remember very little from the first five months after Jack's death. I knew I needed to live in the moment, but it felt as if each day were a distant reach away. Reality was elusive—like extending your hand out as far as possible to find you can only graze the fingertips of a friend falling to his death.

I was simply going through the motions when I returned to the university. However, that semester, it seemed I was a lighthouse for distressed ships. Student after student revealed to me they had depression or bipolar disorder. They told me how they struggled to get up every morning. A couple were hospitalized.

It was a harsh cosmic joke, or a test, I thought, as if the death of my own family member weren't enough. Or maybe I was just more sensitive to the realities of the college world and in tune with the traumas we all suffer. I think I struggled with my capacity to discern when someone was in distress.

One student came to me very late to register for classes. Frustrated after a long day of putting out last-minute fires and by the fact he had not filled out all the necessary forms before he arrived, I snapped, "Please take these forms and bring them back filled out."

He softly apologized. He told me he was legally blind and his mother had completed suicide a week ago. He had to take care of his younger brother because there was no one else at home. He had to get registered for school. He asked me to help him. He said please.

"What was wrong with me?" I thought. I'd sounded like so many of the health care professionals Jack and I had encountered. Was this a test? Was I being challenged?

Detachment was a way to avoid full mental breakdown, but it cut me off from empathy and compassion. I didn't want to be that person. Empathy makes us more real and vulnerable.

My mission shifted in that moment. I knew all I could do was listen—to hold space for them like the final counselor did for Jack.

I tried to find resources for students who were in crisis; I gave them books to read. I cried with them but also tried to give them hope. I told them all they were experienced was temporary.

I tried to be available, unlike most of the health care practitioners Jack and I had encountered.

The students knew nothing about my own situation. I couldn't talk about it—not because I felt ashamed but because it was too fresh and cut too deep—but I could provide them what Jack had needed: an affirmation of their humanity.

* * *

I have begun sharing my story with those who struggle with their own mental health, or those who deeply love someone going through the same experiences Jack and I went through. I hope empathy is my phoenix rising from the rubble. I'm pressed to be kinder, more understanding, and more tolerant.

I began writing this book five months after Jack's death. A friend of mine asked me to attend a "Write Your Book in a Weekend" workshop offered in the town where Jack had made his first attempt. I resisted. Fear of reliving our history left me paralyzed.

I registered for the workshop anyway. The idea I should write a book about this time in our lives took precedence over my own limitations. Jack had dreamed there would be a book, and I felt determined to make that happen. Little did I know, it would become the primary catalyst for my own healing.

Writing from a place of vulnerability has been so very hard but so remarkably important to my healing. I have learned vulnerability is the transparency that allows us to love fully and completely. Of course, we have to know who to trust with that vulnerability, but overall truth is a powerful tool.

I suppose we have to trust people will honor the space from which truth is born. If they don't, then we can only trust they will learn what it is they need to learn from it, and then we move on.

I've learned true love stands on its own. Love doesn't need to depend on anyone or anything else to thrive. True love is unconditional, no strings attached. Any choice we make about our own lives, will always affect others. To unconditionally love someone through their choices is remarkably hard, and there are times when we get hurt or angry with their decisions. But ultimately, it's through the cathartic release of attachment to the outcomes of their decisions that changes us and helps us evolve into better human beings.

Jack fulfilled the words I spoke to him when I gave him the freedom to choose his own path. In all of my humanness, there are days I want to retract those words, but I believe them to be the truth. By making the decisions he made, in the way he made them, he joined the circle of our family.

Far from finally, but finally for this purpose... I learned I can trust. I can trust the Universe to deliver everything I need without fail. When I have earnestly asked for healing, I've heard, "Trust." I have stepped one foot in front of the other, trusting the ground will rise to meet me. There are times I may be concerned because I can't see the next step, but it is my own weakness that makes me blind to that step. The fog rising from my uncertainty obscures the pathway.

Through prayer and meditation, I have been able to stop looking for the next step. It's there. It's always there. We just need to take it.

We are all connected in a way I understood only minimally before this tragic event in my life. We are connected in ways we may never understand in this lifetime. It's why we laugh when we hear a baby's giggle. It's why we cry when we see the magnificence of the ocean. It's why we are consumed when we look into each other's eyes. To trust the Creator of the Universe, we must feel connected.

We are all here to facilitate each other's growth, to help each other become the best version of ourselves we can possibly manifest.

Afterward

ON TO HEALING

AFTER A TRAGIC OCCURRENCE, it may feel like you will never move on. You want to keep the world from moving, to stop the spin, to quell the aching pain. No one can tell you how long your feelings about the loss will last or how you should grieve, but I can tell you if you allow it to, healing will come.

As a young person, I would roll my eyes when my mother said, "Tomorrow is a new day and this too shall pass." I embrace that philosophy now. I understand how true it really is.

While you're immersed in the slurry of emotions, know there will be a day when you can move on. Life will continue.

Moving on to healing doesn't necessarily mean replacing the person you lost. Humans who have been stripped from our lives leave a gaping hole for a long time; one might argue the hole is there forever. However, only *we* can determine how we recover, how we choose to live.

Moving on in this context simply means embracing the flow of life and being open to what it has to offer. We owe that to ourselves and to our families.

* * *

After Jack's death, I thought it would be impossible to overcome and move forward. It was too overwhelming and painful. Now I am happily remarried to a wonderful and functional man who is also on his own journey of loss and healing. My two boys are grown and thriving. I have four more adult children and two beautiful grandchildren in my life, a gift from my new husband.

Life is good. Life is better than I thought it ever could be. I'm happy, and that's all Jack really wanted for me. I believe that deep in my soul.

The healing process is an individual thing, and to profess the way I healed is the best way for everyone else would be ridiculous. However, I can share with you some of the methods or practices that saved me when I thought I could go on no longer. Though I am a teacher of these processes, I found it difficult to apply them to myself in the hardest of times, but when I did, I was better for it.

No one prescription exists, of course, for overcoming such a tragic loss. Nothing can make you heal faster than you are meant to heal. However, I do believe the more resources we have, the better our odds of healing. The more tools we have in our basket, the more likely it is we'll find something that works for us.

In the following sections I share some tools you may find helpful in working through and understanding loss. Some of these tools I gained *before* Jack's death in response to being a caregiver throughout our marriage. Other tools and resources are results of my own learning in the process of caring for someone who is ill, whether mentally, physically, emotionally, or otherwise.

I also share the resources I found as I faced his death and what future lay ahead for the boys and me. These are resources I hope you never need, but they are here if you do.

These resources carried me through the days of healing myself, my children, and others around me. So often, you are the shoulder upon which everyone else leans, and there is so little time for your own healing. Take that time; be gentle with yourself. It's essential to address the pain and trauma before it all takes over your life.

Emotions

After Jack died, I experienced a rainbow of emotions from the time I arose in the morning until I laid my head down at night. Often, it seemed like there was an enormous magnifying glass over each one. When I felt alone, I felt hugely alone. When I felt anger, I felt intense anger. So often I felt if I acknowledged even one of them, they would take my body and mind hostage.

They all seemed exaggerated, sometimes overwhelming, and often ill placed during the day. Sometimes I would cry for what seemed to be no reason. Other times I would be impatient or short-tempered. And then sometimes I would feel nothing at all when I thought I should have.

There is no question it's important to acknowledge our emotions. As I moved through my experiences with Jack, I learned I should just be honest about my emotions and also kind to myself. I acknowledged my stressors and learned to use the tools I needed to address them.

The deep love we have for the person hurting, the one who is experiencing the pain, creates an accompanying sadness that can be hard to manage. Many times, I wanted to trade places with Jack. I remember thinking it might be easier to take his pain on myself than to watch him wrestle with the demons of mental illness. I doubt that would be true, but I thought it often. It's so very hard to watch someone suffering and tell yourself things will get better. Sometimes it's easy and understandable to slip into depression yourself.

Anger and guilt came in alternating waves for me, before and after Jack took his life. Many days began with love and patience but ended with anger, which, for me, led to guilt.

It was a vicious cycle some days. I was angry he had to experience this kind of illness. I was angry *we* were experiencing what seemed to be a permanent disruption in our lives. I felt angry he was putting us through it all, because I was tired, because I felt he wasn't trying—I could go on and on. Following all that anger came guilt—guilt because of how I felt, guilt because of some of the things I had said to him, guilt because I wasn't more patient or because I'd gotten angry that he wasn't there for me.

After Jack's death, I experienced anger because of the choices he made, and then, knowing those choices stemmed from the fact he was not well, I felt guilty again. Through all of this, it was the guilt that wore me down most.

I believe this to be normal. Elisabeth Kübler-Ross wrote wonderful books about loss and grief. I recommend them all. She said, "Guilt is perhaps the most painful companion of death."

I now seek the awe in life. I meditate on the love of the Universe. I meditate on gratitude for who I am and what life offers me. I am gentle with myself. I try to allow all the feelings of sadness, anger, and frustration to run through me without judgment. Some days I'm very successful, others I'm not. Some days are remarkably hard, but it's important for me to push through and allow the authenticity of the emotions to be expressed.

Breathing

Breathing is an autonomic human function. We all breathe. When we're under duress, however, the body prepares for danger. It releases adrenaline and cortisol, which causes the human body to tense and breathe faster and shallower, attempting to quickly get more oxygen to the muscles so we can engage in the fight-or-flight response. Blood is shunted away from the brain to physical systems that can assist. This response is helpful in many short-term situations but can be very harmful to us in the long run.

After many long days of caregiving, I began to realize I was holding my breath. Days of short, shallow breathing under chronic stress lead to frequently pausing my breath. Instead of more oxygen, my lungs begged for more time with the oxygen they did have so they could extract every molecule possible.

Particularly with the chronic, long-term stress of caregiving and the sudden but extended stress of loss, the body begins to break down in ways that we may not comprehend immediately. This can be detrimental to our own mental, physical, spiritual, and emotional health. During my years as a caregiver and after Jack's death, without conscious breathing, I would have been in much worse physical shape than I was.

One of the best tools I learned in dealing with trauma is to consciously and intentionally breathe. There are many conscious breathing techniques; finding a method that works for you is the most important piece of this. If you attempt something that feels unnatural or uncomfortable, then you won't stick with it.

My most important task was to *recognize* the stress each day and *remember* to breathe deeply when I needed it. To do that, I placed sticky notes at work and around the house that simply said, "BREATHE NOW."

I found it so helpful I ordered ten stones engraved with the word "BREATHE" and strategically placed them in my environment. You can still find them in my plants, on my windowsill, next to my bathtub, and even on my refrigerator door.

Diet and Exercise

It's been well documented diet and exercise are essential to leading a happy, healthy life. There, it had to be said.

But before you roll your eyes, and skip this section, consider this. You may only believe diet and exercise are helpful for maintaining a happy, healthy life but they can also be helpful when we are in the heart of the storm.

I believe that diet and exercise are really important, and I put that belief into practice most of the time. But for me, I find these two areas fall by the wayside when stress overwhelms me.

Experts argue this is actually when you should most maintain healthy life habits. However, chronic stressors demotivate most people from engaging in these activities. Exercise and managing a diet are hard to incorporate during these times, I understand. They take time, energy, and discipline, all of which can be short in supply during crisis. If you can, find a physical activity that is cathartic and relieves stress. Stretching to get your circulation going is really helpful. Eat as well as you can. Understandably, some days, it's hard to remember to eat at all.

People like avid, committed runners, bikers, or other athletes should continue their established habits to manage stress, rather than stopping suddenly. But if you're not an athlete, don't feel you have to become one during a time of stress. Just walk around the block a few times or take time to stretch your body.

Be cautious about using alcohol, mind numbing substances, or self-harming activities to ease the pain. So often, when we make choices that are detrimental to our health, it contributes to the overall crisis, and then no one is healthy enough to manage during the tough times.

Think about the flight attendant's safety instructions prior to takeoff. The instructions are to give yourself oxygen before assisting others who are unable to help themselves. How can we have the strength to be caregivers if we are not in a healthy state of mind? While so tempting to quell the screams of painful memories, try to allow yourself to feel and embrace what has happened.

My advice is to do what you can to maintain healthy lifestyle choices in general. Most importantly, try to be understanding with yourself when you aren't able to maintain your regular health practices. Resume those when you're able. Try to relieve yourself from guilt. Additional guilt is not helpful when in crisis

Counseling

When I lost my mother, I learned it's much better to recognize and address any grief and sadness by allowing myself space to heal. I spent the year after her death staying busy and distracted, and then I crashed. While busyness is a coping mechanism in the beginning, it can become very dysfunctional. It's not worth ignoring or deferring the pain long-term. Eventually, our emotional savings account dries up and we're left with nothing to draw from.

In my case, I knew I didn't want long-term pain controlling me and wrecking my life. Yes, it's painful to work through the trauma but it's much more painful to allow trauma to take over and create havoc in other relationships and everyday functioning.

I sought out counseling for a while after my mother died, and again after Jack died. It does help, but I found for me, I had to be willing to do the work. I felt frustrated with regurgitating my pain. I didn't need someone to validate my pain; I needed to move it to a place of healing. I needed to work on something. So, while I do advocate getting assistance understanding your loss, you may need to engage in what I call "active healing" versus what felt like a more "passive" approach.

I asked my counselor to give me some homework so I felt I was actually doing something. He chuckled and said I was doing something. I was processing the pain by retelling the story. I probably was at some level but I needed to feel I was *actually* doing something to relieve the pain.

Many counselors now realize the brain needs a more cognitive healing experience and are becoming certified in areas such as Eye Movement Rapid Desensitization and Reprocessing (EMDR) and forms of cognitive therapy. I have no personal experience with this method. I wish it had been suggested during my counselling sessions. I know many people who have benefitted from it.

Regardless, we all respond differently to various techniques and the amount of time we need to heal varies remarkably.

Self Care

Most of the techniques mentioned above can be classified as self-care; however, caring for yourself may sometimes mean allowing others to care for you. As a caregiver of someone with illness or distress, we get in the mode of neglecting our own self care, whether that's because we believe we aren't worthy of someone else caring for us or we believe we just don't have time. Natural caregivers are comfortable in this role and provide care for not only the one who is ill, but children, pets, extended family and others.

Many of my friends from the healing arts community were quite skillful in massage, Reiki and other healing methods, hypnosis, meditation and etc. Accepting this help was my first challenge, but when I did, it was remarkably beneficial. It was a chance to let someone else work on my pain.

Self-hypnosis downloads also were very helpful. Some people aren't as trusting of these tools, but I found them to be very useful. Mindfulness and deep meditation were helpful alternatives or supplements to medication. Many studies support the use of hypnosis and self-hypnosis as a method for reducing stress and thereby enhancing the healing process for the mind and body. Regardless of method, find some outlet for you to receive rather than constantly give of your time and resources until they are depleted.

Meditation, Prayer, and Stillness

I learned to truly enjoy being still. It's in the quiet moments I can really hear my inner guidance, a still, small voice I personally believe comes from God. Finding this voice is different for everyone. Some people find spiritual connection in nature or in listening to soft or calming music.

It's in the quietness of the moment we can experience true connectedness if we allow ourselves to. It sounds so simple but it's true.

For me, it's important to my sense of self to feel a part of something greater or more collective than just me alone. By being a part of something larger and more powerful than myself, I find myself feeling grateful.

I learned all of the "right" and "wrong" ways to pray in my Southern Baptist upbringing, and then later the "right" and "wrong" ways to meditate in my healing arts practice. Quite honestly, the directions I received initially for both were counterproductive to finding peace within myself. I felt self-conscious and fearful I wasn't doing things "right," so I got lost in the dictates or the perfunctory nature of formal religion. I remember being called on to pray, and rather than feeling comfortable and connected to God, I felt it was a performance—that I would be graded on how well I prayed. That's all changed for me now.

I resolved I don't have to perform "correctly" to feel connected to God. For some, ritual is very comforting and reassuring, but everyone is different. I found I could connect with nature while hiking outdoors and feel God. I didn't need the rules anymore. In the still of the moment, I meditate and focus on gratitude for who I am and how I fit in the world, and not whether I'm in the right stance or perched on the meditation mat appropriately. I pray when I seek help, guidance, or solace, wherever I am.

Finding stillness may not involve meditating or praying for some. It may be that connecting with quietness means just sitting still long enough to sort out the tangles. Or maybe it just helps us hear our inner voice giving us direction. I can be quiet anywhere I am and I don't have to be specifically meditating or praying. Quietness is a way to signal to the brain, "I'm listening now."

So often, we don't want to hear the still voices in our head and heart because it's painful. We may fear the inner voice will reveal a truth we don't want to face. But it's in the quietness our subconscious mind can speak to us, helping us through the pain. If we stay so busy we cannot hear that still, small voice, then the solutions to our pain have greater difficulty reaching us.

I believe by being a part of the magnificence of all that is, I am by default part of the magnificence of the Universe. It's a great confidence builder and it's a relief I'm not ultimately the one in control of my life. Thank goodness! There are days when I can really muck things up!

When I intentionally seek quietness, I find a place where I can close a door. When I had young children, some days I would retreat to the bathroom. Now, perched upon the side of the bathtub, in the shower, in my bedroom, or behind a door in my office, I close my eyes and check in with my body.

I take three to five really deep breaths, and depending on my level of stress, I may hold it for a few seconds in between.

I ask myself quietly how I am feeling. Where am I holding my stress, pain, anger, or other emotions? How do I feel when I don't have those feelings? I ask myself how I can best address these emotions in the short term (to get through the day) or long term (usually entailing more work).

Then I sit in the quiet of a few short minutes, and I listen to whatever messages come through. If nothing concrete comes, then I thank myself for the break and invariably I feel I can better continue my day.

Affirmations

Sometimes it's helpful to create affirmations. These are simply encouraging, positive messages for yourself, such as "I have a great smile" or "I'm a good friend." You may even take it a step further and remind yourself something like, "I am happy, I have enough, and I am enough," or "I'm strong enough to make it through this day."

I created a bowl of affirmations I kept on my desk at work. I found I wasn't the only one who needed them; so did my colleagues, who would stop by my office to pick one out of the bowl now and then.

Affirmations are probably similar to adages you've heard in your own family. My mother would say things like "This too shall pass" or "Early to bed and early to rise makes a man healthy, wealthy, and wise." Humanity has created adages of all kinds and in many walks of life, and like affirmations, they're meant to encourage us, to give us hope for a positive outcome. The same impulse to connect with these truths is why we love the fortune cookies we get at Chinese restaurants. Relishing their words of encouragement and inspiration, we tuck them away in our pockets for safekeeping.

Find affirmations that work for you. It can be very helpful to repeat them as you sit in the quiet. Maybe write them on cards and leave them around in your environment so you can read them throughout the day. Go out on a limb and even write phrases like "I am love" or "I deserve love," or maybe "My challenges are simply gifts to make me stronger and wiser." Make them believable, even if they are hard to conceive in the present situation.

Music

I found music that lowered my heart rate helpful, especially when I felt stress and anxiety getting control of me. Music is so healing anyway.

Find music that calms you or nurtures rather than agitates you. Generally, studies demonstrate music that is closely aligned with nature or the biological systems of humans is best overall. For example, music that corresponds with human heart rates has been found to be more healing. Instrumentals or classical music can do the same. Hospitals are implementing programs using music postoperatively.

I downloaded a type of music for Jack and myself research has found to be useful in managing stress, mental health conditions, and other healing. It's called Hemi-Sync, but many other types of music can serve the same purpose; meditation music is another good option. Find what works best for you or your loved ones.

Empathy

Empathy is different from sympathy and much more difficult to achieve.

The days I felt sympathy for Jack I felt sorry for him or, even worse, I pitied him. I treated him like a child, which contributed to the inordinate and degrading pain he felt. That was unfair to him and created a deep resentment in me I didn't need.

Sympathy required no understanding of Jack. Empathy did.

Empathy is a hard emotion to capture when your loved one is experiencing pain or feelings you have never felt. Some would argue it's impossible to understand.

Some days, caring for Jack felt like an act of love, but I found it to be trying when exhaustion set in, or the utter frustration when he seemed to give up though I wanted him to keep trying. These were the days when I felt my burden increased exponentially and I felt very alone in the struggle.

Those days, I closed my eyes and tried to imagine what it would be like to walk in his shoes. What would it be like to feel the way he felt? How difficult must it be to feel that kind of depression and dysfunction?

It was hard. Many days, I may not have been good at it, but on the days that I was able to muster empathy, I was kinder, I was more loving, and I renewed my commitment to what I felt was keeping him alive.

Once he was gone, I tried to understand how it must have felt to want to give in and give up. I imagined how it must have felt to be in that much pain every day. I tried so hard to understand why he made the choices he made.

While I still felt angry, I believe this empathy helped expedite my healing process because I was able to forgive. The act of forgiving requires the compassion to understand another person. And in that understanding, we can forgive him or her.

So, is it that easy?

Of course it isn't, but it's a place to start.

While I never completely understood what Jack was feeling, I *can* understand he felt he was too sick to stay. I *can* understand he truly loved us and he couldn't bear to put us through what life would have been like with his illness long-term. I *can* understand he was in so much pain he just couldn't live any longer. It's through seeking to understand we can eventually forgive, and through forgiving we can begin to heal.

* * *

Jack's dream told me what to write in this book. He said it would be about our experiences, so others could know they aren't alone, and it would help people heal from loss. My sincerest hope is the process of revisiting our story will be helpful to others who read this book; however, the cathartic writing of the last five years has facilitated my own healing. For that I am grateful.

The flow of life rocks us to the core when we feel we cannot endure it. Unjustly shaking the boat are the tumultuous storms of time, the violent winds of change, and the fractured drought of loss. Each of these can break us or build us. The decision is assuredly ours to make.

Acknowledgments

THANK YOU ISN'T ADEQUATE enough to express my deep indebtedness for those who were there in the depths of my despair and recovery. My family, particularly my brother and sister-in-law, father, and boys gave me the strength to push through each day.

Friends are extensions to our strength when we feel our strength has run out. I am eternally grateful for the friends who stood by me in the darkest hours.

It's so important to feel we aren't alone. And I wasn't.

About the Author

D. R. FREDI Ph.D. has a passion for assisting families experiencing mental health, trauma and suicide. After 20 years worth of experience working with people who experienced war trauma, she found herself dealing with her own family crisis.

Diagnosed bipolar, her late husband tried multiple times to take his life, ultimately resulting in his death from a completed suicide. His illness and their journey together challenged her every skill as a Public Health practitioner and as a human being.

Grappling with how to heal from her own trauma, she shares her story in hopes that it may help even one person heal from the loss of a loved one. She lives happily remarried and re-engaged in life and living to help others through the loss of their loved ones.

Visit www.SuicideFree.org for more resources, to build community, and support each other in recovery.

Please take the time to leave a review on Amazon to spread awareness of this book and resources.

www.SuicideFree.org